Addiction Private Practice

The Definitive Guide for Addiction
Counselors and Therapists

Michael O'Brien, CADC II, NCAC I

Contents

Foreword

Michael O'Brien and I share a core value: a commitment to helping counselors succeed in their alcohol and drug counseling careers. Michael's book, *Addiction Private Practice - Second Edition*, continues to support substance abuse counselors as they venture into private practice. I wish I had access to such are source when I began my journey decades ago. Upon reviewing this book, I am impressed by how thoroughly Michael addresses all the nuances of private practice.

Alcohol and drug counselors often enter private practice with substantial knowledge of the field and years of counseling experience. However, traditional training programs seldom cover the "business" aspects of running a private practice. Michael sheds light on this subject like no other. Having spent decades in private practice, I learned to manage my practice through "on-the-job training," making many mistakes along the way. I even considered pursuing an MBA at one point but did not. My greatest challenges in private practice involved personnel issues, handling paperwork, and dealing with insurance and audits. I highly recommend following Michael's advice to alleviate these common headaches.

In the 1990s, I wrote *Global Criteria: The 12 Core Functions of the Substance Abuse Counselor* to help new counselors understand their daily and weekly responsibilities. My goal was to prepare them for both the oral and written examinations, essential steps in advancing their careers. During training sessions on the 12 Core Functions, I always emphasized that my training would not ensure passing the examination but would help competent counselors demonstrate their competence. As you consider entering private practice, use available resources to ease the transition. Learn from others' experiences; learn from Michael what works.

Michael's guide for addiction counselors and therapists transitioning into private practice is a treasure trove of ideas, processes, and resources designed for your success. I suggest reading and re-reading the material in this book. Albert Einstein, who I believe was quite intelligent, once remarked that he didn't know everything but knew where to find answers. Be as smart as Einstein.

John W. Herdman, Ph.D.

Author of *Global Criteria: The 12 Core Functions of the Substance Abuse Counselor-8th Edition*.

CEO of HerdmanHealth

www.herdmanhealth.com

Preface

Introduction to the Updated Edition

Almost five years have passed since I published the first edition of my book. In that short time, the world has undergone significant changes. The COVID-19 pandemic had a dramatic effect on telehealth, leading to a radical acceptance of this service delivery method that is unprecedented. While there will always be a need for inpatient and residential services, telehealth has provided more opportunities for flexibility, improving income, and helping more people than we ever imagined.

The pandemic also ushered in an era of unprecedented mortality rates from substance abuse and suicide. The opioid epidemic continues unabated, with overdose deaths reaching new records. There has never been a more urgent need for qualified and compassionate professionals in our field. The workforce needs in substance use disorder treatment are immense across the nation and pay levels in treatment programs and rates in private practice have never been higher.

Though my book caters to a niche sector of the behavioral health workforce. The number of people who have read *Addiction Private Practice* has surprised me. I know that hundreds, if not thousands, of additional substance use disorder professionals are in private practice today compared to five years ago. I am proud to call many of you my friends. It continues to be the book that recovery programs don't want you to read. I've updated the content and tools and expanded it to include information on telehealth and other important topics.

If you haven't done so yet, stop what you are doing and visit A ddictionPrivatePractice.com to explore the resources now available to you. Thank you for purchasing this book. I sincerely appreciate your support and look forward to working with you as you start your journey in private practice.

The Impact of Our Work

There are few careers where one can have such a significant impact on society. Every time someone becomes clean and sober, a ripple effect occurs. Their relationships improve, they become better parents and employees, there are fewer emergency room visits, and healthcare expenses are reduced. Arrests, legal issues, and incarceration decrease significantly, as do accidents, sick days, and premature deaths. The positive effects are staggering and so significant that it is difficult for us to see their full impact. I feel this positive impact and a strong sense of purpose every day I do this work. I've found my calling, and I feel it in every session with my clients. I hope you can do the same by utilizing this book.

Behavioral health professionals in private practice can effectively treat mild-to-moderate substance use disorders. Those severe enough to need residential treatment would have more opportunities to receive it if lower-severity clients filled fewer beds. We are simply not doing enough to provide options and remove barriers to treatment for people with mild-to-moderate substance use disorders. People with mild disorders often progress to severe disorders because they do not feel that the options are appropriate for problems at their end of the spectrum. Addiction professionals in private practice fill a critical need for individuals considering addressing their substance use before it becomes moderate or severe.

Halfway through my career as an addiction professional, I became severely disillusioned and was prepared to exit the field entirely. Inefficient, ineffective, and dysfunctional are just a few words to describe the state of many treatment programs. To make matters worse, the cost of living in California has been skyrocketing for decades. Even a position that pays $25 per hour would still be less than poverty-level wages. I asked myself, "Is there a way I can help others and make an income I can survive on?" The answer was—maybe. Perhaps it would be possible for me to achieve these goals in private practice? There was no way to be sure. After confirming with my certifying agency, I could see clients in a private office setting. I set out to do just that. This journey in addiction private practice has made me happier and more successful than I could have ever imagined. I've written this book so that you can achieve or exceed my success.

While I've written this book for addiction counselors, the business practices outlined within can work for other behavioral health professionals anywhere in the United States. I'm sharing with you the blueprint for my success. You must be certain that you have the qualifications necessary to do this work in your jurisdiction. If you do not, you may hurt the people you are trying to help, lose your career, and possibly lose your freedom.

When I started my practice, I searched for books, seminars, guides—anything about how to start and run an addiction practice. I found zero resources. Not one colleague or any of the people I went to school with were in private practice. Many left the field for the exact reasons I outlined previously. I felt I was entering uncharted waters. I was uncertain whether I could attract clients, how many clients I would have, or what my income would be. Am I the first addiction counselor to start a private practice? No, there have been others before me. It just felt like I was the first one.

If you can make it through the expense, education, internships, dysfunctional coworkers, borderline clients, and intense treatment environments, along with all the difficulties in becoming an addiction counselor, you can succeed—no, you can thrive — in private practice. There is nothing more complicated about private practice than becoming an addiction counselor. You've survived the gauntlet, the industry, and the people. Private practice is your opportunity to self-actualize, earn the income you deserve, and effectively help more people.

You don't need to understand how to use every tool, service, or process I explain in this book immediately. Set them up and start using them! You will gain competence as you use them. Take advantage of the additional training and support I've set up at AddictionP rivatePractice.com. Eventually, you will master this, and everything you've learned will become second nature. If we had to understand everything precisely the way it worked, every time we used something, we would get nothing done. You wouldn't start your car because you don't know how a combustion engine works. You'd never turnon a light switch because you don't understand how electricity works. We take leaps of faith every day. This one can truly set you free.

I have already tried all the things that didn't work, were too expensive, too complicated, or completely wasted my time. I've made most of the mistakes for you. I've also proven that competent and compassionate addiction professionals can thrive in private practice and save lives both safely and ethically. Have faith in yourself. I have faith in you. Follow the steps and suggestions in this book. Don't skip any steps or leave anything out. Take the leap of faith and find your success in private practice.

While I provide a streamlined and efficient business model in this book, my goal was not to teach the clinical aspects of how to perform things like screening, assessment, counseling, and other core functions. Instead, it is to teach you the process in which I carry them out. I will launch additional training on how to master these critical core functions in the future.

Thank you for the life-saving work that you do. I look forward to seeing many of you exceed my accomplishments and success. Together, *we* are changing the world!

Michael O'Brien, CADC II, NCAC I

Chapter One

Everything You
Need to Succeed

C ongratulations on taking the first step towards running a successful private practice!

I wrote this book to give you a thorough understanding of what it
takes to operate a thriving private practice. While it contains a lot of
critical information, there is simply too much to include in one book.

Addictionprivatepractice.com, is a comprehensive resource packed
with everything you need for your private practice. On the website,
you'll find in-depth articles that expand on the topics in this book,
along with new insights and tools that I started using after publication.
There are courses, downloadable forms, and a wealth of additional
resources to support your journey.

Unlocking the Power of Marketing

One of the most daunting aspects of running a private practice is marketing. If you're like me, you probably find marketing intimidating

and time consuming. That's why I developed a proprietary marketing system that simplifies the entire process. This system is so valuable that I couldn't include it in the book, but it's available on the website. It's the best way to attract new clients quickly, without the usual hassle.

Join a Thriving Community

You don't have to do this alone. On our website, you can join a community of like-minded professionals who are also starting and thriving in their private practices. Connect with others on the same journey, share tips, ideas, and challenges, and find the support you need. It's a great place to make friends and get inspired.

Leave a Review

If you find this book helpful, please consider leaving a review on Amazon. Reviews are crucial for the success of any book on Amazon, and your feedback will help others who want to start their own practice. Together, we can help thousands of additional clients by spreading the word.

Stay Connected

For more information and ongoing support, follow me on social media:

X (Twitter): https://x.com/addictionpp

Facebook: https://www.facebook.com/addictionprivatepractice

Instagram: https://www.instagram.com/addictionprivatepractice/

LinkedIn: https://www.linkedin.com/company/addictionprivat epractice/

Threads: https://www.threads.net/@addictionprivatepractice

YouTube: https://www.youtube.com/@addictionprivatepractice

Thank you, again. I am incredibly excited to begin this journey with you. I look forward to seeing you online.

Chapter Two

Scope of Practice and Terminology

I have placed this information in the first chapter of my book because it provides essential guidance for those starting a private practice as substance use disorder (SUD) counselors.

As a mental health professional, such as a licensed psychologist, licensed professional clinical counselor (LPCC), or licensed marriage and family therapist (LMFT), you can legally offer all the services discussed in this book in most states. Similarly, if you hold a license as a substance use disorder professional, you can offer these services in most jurisdictions. If you are a certified SUD professional without state licensing, your ability to offer these services depends on your state's specific laws and regulations.

Regulations for SUD professionals vary significantly across states and are continually evolving. Some states license SUD professionals, some only offer certification, and others provide both with different scopes of practice. Certain states only certify SUD counselors and restrict them from private practice, while others allow it. It is crucial to verify that your credentials permit you to practice in a private office setting. Understanding and adhering strictly to your scope of practice is essential. Non-compliance may result in severe consequences, including the loss of your career and personal freedom.

Using the correct terminology for your license or certification level is also crucial. Psychologists and therapists have a broader range of terms to describe or advertise their services. Certified SUD professionals should exercise caution and should only use a limited range of acceptable terminology to describe or advertise their services. Certified counselors should use the exact credential type listed on their certification. For example, as a CADC II or NCAC I, you can use "Certified Alcohol & Drug Counselor" or "National Certified Addiction Counselor." Using incorrect or misleading titles can be unethical and possibly illegal.

The public often struggles to understand the various credentials and what they mean. It is your responsibility to help them comprehend your qualifications. Correct and educate clients, other professionals, or members of the public if they use incorrect terminology or misunderstand your credentials.

I often receive communications from prospective clients addressed to "Dr. O'Brien." When this happens, I promptly correct them, saying, "I noticed you called me Dr. O'Brien on your voicemail. I wanted to clarify that I'm an SUD counselor, not a physician. I cannot prescribe medication or treat medical conditions. Do you have questions about my credentials or my scope of practice?" When you correct or educate a client, it is essential to note this information in their file.

Advertising or referring to your services as therapy or medical treatment is illegal if you are not licensed to provide these services. Clients are the individuals receiving care from counselors, not patients. As SUD counselors, we provide aftercare, assessments, consultation, counseling, drug testing, education, evaluations, interventions, referrals, and screening. The terminology used to describe our field varies by location and includes terms such as alcohol or drug counseling, substance abuse counseling, drug abuse counseling, chemical dependency counseling, substance use disorder counseling, and addiction counseling.

Correcting clients, other professionals, or members of the public may feel uncomfortable, but I have never lost a client by being honest and transparent. This fear of losing clients is likely the reason some SUD professionals misrepresent their credentials. Clients appreciate clarity, and it sets a crucial first impression that the relationship will operate within appropriate ethical boundaries. Many clients have previously seen providers with higher credentials without success and are looking for someone with your unique experience and expertise. Demonstrating integrity and honesty from the outset is essential. If you haven't reviewed your scope of practice or code of conduct recently, do so before launching your practice. Visit your certifying or licensing board's website to ensure you have the latest version.

Chapter Three

Services Provided in Private Practice

S tarting a private practice requires careful consideration of the services you will offer within your scope of practice. This chapter outlines the services commonly provided by substance use disorder (SUD) professionals in private practice. We will briefly discuss each service here, and later in the book, we will cover the steps required to deliver each service effectively.

Common Services:

- Aftercare Counseling and Relapse Prevention

- Standard Alcohol and Drug Assessments

- Third-Party Alcohol and Drug Assessments

- Alcohol and Drug Counseling

- Alcohol and Drug Education

- Consultation Services

- Drug Testing and Monitoring

- Group Alcohol and Drug Counseling

- Interventions

- Treatment Placement Assistance

- SAP/SAE Services

Aftercare Counseling and Relapse Prevention

Clients who have completed an inpatient or outpatient treatment program often need ongoing aftercare support. These sessions reinforce the tools and strategies learned during treatment and introduce additional techniques. Critical components include educating the client, implementing relapse prevention strategies, and providing ongoing support as the client navigates early recovery.

Standard Alcohol and Drug Assessments

A comprehensive assessment is the cornerstone of the counseling relationship and is crucial for client success. In my practice, I use the **Herdman Assessment Form (HAF)** for substance use disorders. This thorough process results in a personalized recovery plan or referrals to more appropriate clinicians or higher levels of care. Every new client, and those seeking treatment placement help, must undergo this assessment. To ensure suitability for the level of care and within my scope of practice, I must re-evaluate clients who are returning after a break of over thirty days.

This assessment is one of the most time-intensive services offered. It involves:

Administration of Assessment Tools: Using the HAF

Documentation: Recording detailed client information.

Narrative Writing: Summarizing findings and insights.

Creation and Discussion of a Recovery Plan: Developing a tailored plan for each client.

In the past, this process could take three to four hours. However, with experience and tools like the HAF, you can complete this process more efficiently in about 90-minutes. Because of the time and effort involved, I charge a higher rate for assessments.

For many providers, the most time-consuming parts of the assessment process are documentation, narrative writing, and scoring. Fortunately, tools like the assessment software available at Herdman-Health can make these tasks quicker and easier. Some of the key features include:

Electronic Versions of the ASI and ASI Lite: These digital tools save significant time and streamline the assessment process.

Automated Scoring and Documentation: Reduce the manual workload, allowing you to focus more on client care.

Comprehensive Resource Hub: Access in-depth articles, courses, and additional tools to support your practice.

By utilizing these tools, you can enhance your efficiency, ensure thorough assessments, and ultimately provide better care for your clients.

Third-Party Alcohol and Drug Assessments

Third-party assessments are evaluations required or reviewed by a third party. These assessments can involve the following scenarios:

- Judges in criminal court requesting an evaluation for sentencing

- Spouses seeking an assessment because of marital issues

- Physicians requiring an evaluation for patients with early refills or lost prescriptions

- Sports organizations needing an assessment for players with suspected substance abuse issues

- DMV requiring an assessment to reinstate a driver's license after a DUI

- Parents requiring an adult child to undergo an assessment

- Family Court requesting an assessment of a parent accused of a substance use disorder

- Drug Dependency Court requesting an assessment of a parent who may have a substance use disorder

Clients in these scenarios might be less transparent, requiring additional steps: lab-verified drug tests, reviews of police reports, court transcripts, and collateral contacts. These assessments involve a delicate balance of providing a fair report that helps the client address their SUD issues while allowing the third party to make informed decisions. Due to the extra components, I charge a higher rate for third-party assessments. Always review documentation from the requesting party before agreeing to complete the evaluation to ensure you are qualified to conduct it.

Two types of third-party assessments are extremely high risk for certified SUD counselors: family court cases and drug dependency court cases. Family courts handling divorce and custody proceedings often request assessments for parents accused of having an SUD. Similarly, drug dependency courts actively seek assessments for parents whose ability to parent safely is questioned because of an SUD. These cases are high stakes for any parent involved, and those who lose custody will often attempt every legal maneuver available to discredit you and your work. These types of cases have the highest rate of malpractice claims. If you are a certified-only professional, it is best to leave this work to licensed professionals such as psychologists, LMFTs, and LCSWs.

Alcohol and Drug Counseling

I offer counseling sessions in thirty-minute, forty-five-minute, and sixty-minute durations. The sessions focus on achieving the objectives of the recovery plan. Sessions also include additional time for charting. Depending on the client's initial presentation, I might start with multiple weekly sessions until the client stabilizes, then taper the frequency over time as the client progresses in their recovery.

Alcohol and Drug Education

Educational sessions, often required by courts or educational institutions, cover various topics such as the effects of substance abuse and responsible use. Education sessions can also be helpful for family members who need to better understand substance use disorders.

Consultation Services

Consultation services provide information or education to resolve substance abuse-related issues. Examples include family members concerned about a loved one's use, parents exploring treatment options for a student, or clients seeking second opinions on previous assessments. Most consultation sessions are a single visit.

Drug Testing and Monitoring

While I do not require clients to undergo drug tests as a standard policy, there are scenarios where drug testing is necessary or requested. Clients who require legally defensible tests are referred to a laboratory and may need a prescription to have these tests covered by insurance.

Family Education Sessions

Although I do not provide family counseling, I do offer family education sessions. These sessions help family members understand the client's disorder, how they can support recovery, and establish new boundaries or trust. If ongoing family system issues arise, I refer clients to licensed marriage and family therapists while continuing individual counseling.

Group Counseling

Group counseling can be highly effective in private practice when participants are engaged and willing. Once your practice grows, forming specialty groups for women, men, young adults, or specific professions can be beneficial. Specialty certifications for working with subgroups like LGBTQ+ communities, first responders, and others are also available.

Interventions

Interventions can be full-scale family interventions, which are time-consuming and costly, or office interventions where the substance user is aware of the meeting in advance and consents to take part. I provide office interventions but refer full-scale interventions to specialists because of time involved in full-scale interventions.

Treatment Placement Assistance

Assisting clients in finding appropriate treatment options is a valuable service, especially given the abundance of misinformation online. I maintain relationships with withdrawal management facilities and treatment programs across the country. While my client is at a program, I follow up to ensure quality care. It is essential to provide referrals to free or low-cost options for clients who cannot afford your services. Accepting compensation for referral from the provider who will treat the client, also known as "kick backs," is unethical and often illegal.

SAP/SAE Services

Substance Abuse Professional (SAP) and Substance Abuse Expert (SAE) designations, created by the Department of Transportation (DOT) and Nuclear Regulatory Commission (NRC), allow you to protect public safety and generate additional income. These roles involve serious responsibilities, and becoming an SAP or SAE can be rewarding. You can find more information regarding becoming an SAP or SAE on the AddictionPrivatePractice.com website.

This chapter has summarized the various services offered by SUD professionals in private practice. You have the freedom to offer multiple services or focus on specific ones you enjoy. If you intend to provide counseling services, offering assessment services is crucial, as effective counseling begins with a thorough assessment. Later in the book, we will explore how to provide these services in greater detail. For now, decide which services you intend to offer so we can determine the infrastructure, equipment, and supplies for your practice.

Chapter Four

Understanding Your Vision and Income

T his chapter will help you answer the following questions:
- What will your transition to private practice look like?

- What will your schedule look like?

- What is your desired monthly income?

Transitioning to Private Practice

There are two common scenarios when starting a practice:

Gradual Transition: If you have a job, I recommend not quitting immediately. The safest transition is to start your practice while still employed and leave your current position once you have enough clients to replace your income. Some counselors reach a certain income level and then leave their job entirely, while others switch to part-time or contract positions and continue their roles alongside their practice.

Immediate Transition: If you are unemployed, or stuck in a toxic work environment, you may wish to launch your practice as quickly as possible.

Regardless of your transition type, you will gain new clients at a similar rate, and start-up costs will be comparable. I will teach you how to keep your monthly expenses to a minimum later in this book.

Building Your Client Base

Most new practices gain clients gradually rather than experiencing a sudden influx. Slowly ramping up to your ideal client load is beneficial because it allows you to refine your tools and processes, preparing you for more clients and a comfortable workflow.

I have created a proprietary marketing method for professionals in private practice, a game-changer, that eliminates the need for traditional, time-consuming, and anxiety-inducing marketing activities like cold calling and networking. It is simply too valuable to include in this book. However, I will cover standard marketing techniques. With this advanced system, you can effortlessly attract new clients and fill your practice within a few months. This revolutionary approach work for everyone, regardless of their marketing experience, making it accessible and highly effective. The comprehensive marketing course, too valuable to include in my book, is only available on Addiction PrivatePractice.com. Transform your practice with ease and focus on what you do best—helping your clients.

Planning Your Schedule

Here are some things to consider when planning your schedule:

- **Evening Hours**: These are more popular because people prefer not to leave work.

- **Weekend Hours**: I have found that fewer clients prefer services on the weekend. Most people like to keep their weekends free. However, you will still be able to attract clients on the weekend if you are transitioning and working full time during the week.

For example, if you work on Mondays and Tuesdays from 8 a.m. to 10 a.m., you will probably have fewer clients than if you work from 5 p.m. to 7 p.m. More convenient appointment times attract more clients and lead to faster growth.

Sample Initial Schedule:

- Saturdays, 10 a.m. to 5 p.m. (7 hours)

- Sundays, 12 p.m. to 5 p.m. (5 hours)

- **Total client hours per week**: 12

- **Total client hours per month**: 48

Schedule for One Year:

- Mondays, 11 a.m. to 7 p.m. (8 hours)

- Tuesdays, 11 a.m. to 7 p.m. (8 hours)

- Wednesdays, 11 a.m. to 7 p.m. (8 hours)

- Thursdays, 11 a.m. to 7 p.m. (8 hours)

- **Total client hours per week**: 32

- **Total client hours per month**: 128

Setting Fees

While we will discuss setting your fees in more detail later, let's assume the following for now:

- **Counseling**: $100 per hour

- **Standard assessment**: $200 each

- **Third-party assessment**: $400 each

- **Drug test**: $30 each

Calculating Potential Income

Initial Schedule:

- 5 counseling sessions (60 minutes each) = $500

- 1 standard assessment = $200

- 2 drug tests = $60

- **Weekly revenue**: $760

- **Monthly revenue**: $3,040

- **Annual revenue**: $36,480

One Year Schedule:

- 23 counseling sessions (60 minutes each) = $2,300

- 2 standard assessments = $400

- 1 third-party assessment = $400

- 7 drug tests = $210

- **Weekly revenue**: $3,310

- **Monthly revenue**: $13,240

- **Annual revenue**: $158,880

Managing Workload and Income

The maximum number of clients a counselor can see in a week varies, but the full one-year schedule listed above is about the maximum one person can handle safely and effectively. Thirty-one hours of sessions and several assessments each week will keep you very busy. It will also make you financially successful and enable you to help more people than you ever imagined.

Before calculating a budget based on $13,240 per month, remember that you will need to deduct taxes, expenses, and other costs. Assuming expenses total 40% of your gross monthly revenue, or $5,296, your net monthly income would be $7,944. We will cover taxes, expenses, and other costs in more detail later in this book.

Private Practice is Empowering

Knowing how many days and hours per week you want to work and your target income is crucial. With proper planning, you can achieve an income of $180,000 per year with a more intense schedule or higher rates. The work feels much less stressful than other positions I've held in treatment programs. When you set your schedule, avoid dealing with a dysfunctional organization or coworkers, and work with clients who want to make positive changes, the magic happens. You don't feel exhausted with a heavy schedule because you're empowered and excited.

Chapter Five

Setting Your Fees: Valuing Your Expertise

S etting your fees is a crucial step before starting your practice. It reflects the value of your time, experience, education, and expertise. If you don't value yourself, no one else will. Many counselors struggle with properly valuing their services. Besides understanding your worth, it's essential to consider the socioeconomic status of the area where you will be practicing.

Fees for counseling services vary widely by location. A clinician in rural Montana will command a lower hourly rate than one in Beverly Hills, California. This disparity isn't due to one clinician being better than the other; it's because the cost of doing business in Beverly Hills is significantly higher. Prospective clients in most rural areas have lower incomes compared to those in urban areas.

A common mistake counselors make is setting their fees too low. Initially, many are comfortable with a pricing structure that is much lower than what they should be charging. When I started my office in Silicon Valley, one of the most prosperous and expensive places in the country, I charged $80 per hour. This amount seemed terrific, especially after making less than $25 an hour in most programs. A psychologist friend advised me, "You should charge what I charge and see what happens." She was charging $200 per hour. My initial reaction was adverse—I thought, "There's no way someone will pay an addiction counselor $200 for an hour of substance abuse counseling." Fortunately, I moved past that fear. While I didn't set my rate at $200 per hour, I set it at $150 per hour. My friend was right! After a few months, I had more clients than I ever dreamed possible. At $80 per hour, my monthly revenue would have been $9,600, which I thought was acceptable. Instead, by charging $150, my income was $18,000.

Previously in my career, I had never been in a position where I had to ask a client for money. I didn't want my clients to feel like I was in it for the money, and asking for payment felt awkward and made me anxious. However, I realized that all professionals, such as attorneys, dentists, doctors, and massage therapists, ask for their fees. I also learned that when clients feel they are getting excellent results from their sessions, they are happy to pay for your services. Addiction counselors can charge anywhere from $50 to $200 per hour, depending on where they practice. So, what will you charge? Here's a straightforward exercise to help you determine your rate:

1. Go to PsychologyToday.com.

2. Click on "Find a Therapist" on the front page and type in the zip code where you intend to practice.

3. Click on "Addiction" on the left side of the screen. This will show all the clinicians in this directory who advertise under addiction in your zip code.

4. If you see any clinicians with your credentials, click on their name and then click on the button for their website. You should be able to find their rates on their website. If you can't find a clinician with the same certifications or license, choose an LMFT.

5. Calculate the average hourly rate by adding the hourly rates of five providers in your area and dividing the total by five.

That is your new hourly rate. Don't overthink the rate; just accept it for now. This is the rate you will charge per hour for services. If this number feels too high, it is probably the right number. Remember, you can always lower your rates if you run into trouble, but raising them too quickly can cause problems.

Chapter Six

Sliding Scale and Pro Bono Services

When starting out, many counselors have a tendency to offer a sliding scale or reduced rates to lower-income clients. This is often due to:

- A desire to help people and guilt about turning away those who can't afford services.

- The need to build a caseload rapidly when starting with no clients.

- Familiarity with sliding scales from previous agency work.

However, I recommend against offering a sliding scale or reduced rates for several reasons:

- If clients know others are paying less, it can cause dissatisfaction.

- Applying the sliding scale unfairly across all clients is unethical.

- It complicates billing and takes more time to manage.

- Insurance companies dislike clients having different rates, or paying more than others, for the same services.

- Charging insurance companies more than private-pay clients can lead to serious billing issues.

- Clients who pay less often take up more of your time.

Consider the 80/20 rule: 20% of your clients will take up 80% of your time. These 20% are usually the clients paying lower fees. Clients paying higher fees are often more conscious of the time they use. Counselors may resent clients who pay less and take up more time, which can affect client care. I have found that clients who pay out of pocket are more engaged, wanting to realize more value for their money.

Instead of offering a sliding scale, consider offering shorter appointment times. Clients can opt for thirty-minute sessions if that suits their budget. Thirty-minute sessions can be just as effective as one-hour sessions. You can even offer two thirty-minute sessions per month for clients who need them. This flexibility allows you to help more people.

Pro Bono Clients

Some counselors take on several pro bono (completely free) clients per month. If you decide to offer pro bono services, set clear guidelines that apply equally to all clients. You should establish a specific income requirement and verify their income. Develop a waiting list for pro bono clients to manage availability and demonstrate fairness. Documenting when clients decline services ensures your process remains ethical and transparent.

Chapter Seven

Start-Up Costs and Budget

B efore setting up your practice, let's review the start-up costs. Starting out is much less expensive than you might think. Here are the approximate start-up costs for most counselors who follow the suggestions in this book:

Furnished Office Space $400.00

Phone Number $0

Domain Name $15.00

Email Address $20.00

Malpractice Insurance $175

Professional Headshot $250

Website $40

Directory Profiles $300

Business Cards $30

Client Forms $49.99 (on AddictionPrivatePractice.com)

EHR System $100

Business License $100

Legal Structure $150

Drug Tests $100

Total Costs: $1,730

Did you ever imagine you could start your dream business for less than $1,800? It is possible. These are approximate expenses and may vary depending on your location, but most counselors should expect to spend close to these amounts. The highest variable cost is your office space, which we will discuss later.

The cost of starting your practice is so low that most counselors can afford to start right away with their own money. You will probably be able to cover your ongoing monthly expenses with just one client. It's rare to find another legitimate business opportunity with such low start-up costs, high-income potential, and a significant impact on the world.

Chapter Eight

Insurance Billing vs. Private Pay

Out-of-Network (OON) Provider Status

When you start as a counselor, you will automatically be an Out-of-Network (OON) provider. This means you are not part of any insurance company's network. No one starts their practice with the ability to automatically bill insurance as an in-network provider. To become in-network, you must apply, be credentialed (approved) by the insurance company, and sign a contract. This process can take four to twelve months or more for each insurance network you join. "Joining an insurance panel" is another term used to refer to being an in-network provider.

Eligibility for Becoming an In-Network Provider

Licensed clinicians with a master's degree or higher can become in-network providers with nearly every insurance company. Even if you are certified only or have less than a master's degree, you might still have the opportunity to become an in-network provider, depending on the insurance carrier and their requirements. Major changes in this area have occurred in the past few years. Just because you want to join a network doesn't mean they are accepting new providers. You may find that some insurance networks are closed to new providers in some areas where there is over saturation. With time, they will open their network again, check back regularly.

Deciding to Become an In-Network Provider

Everyone starts as an OON provider, allowing you to remain a private-pay counselor and choose to go in-network if you cannot attract enough private-pay clients. In most areas, there are more than enough clients seeking services, so many clinicians never need to accept insurance. I recommend starting your practice as an OON provider and only going in-network if necessary.

Financial Considerations

Insurance companies typically reimburse less per visit than the rate you would charge private-pay clients. For example, if your private-pay rate is $125 per hour but as an in-network provider you receive only $70 per hour, you are losing potential income. However, if you cannot attract enough clients at $125 per visit, then $70 per visit can be beneficial. Most counselors determine within the first six months whether they need to accept insurance to attract sufficient clients. Accepting insurance also lists you in the insurance company's provider directory, which often provides a steady stream of clients. I always like to tell counselors $70 per hour is better than $0. You must decide what rate you are comfortable with.

Cash Flow Challenges

Your immediate cash flow will slow down if you accept insurance. When you accept insurance in-network, you will only receive co-pays from your clients, and there will be a gap of thirty to ninety days before you receive regular payments from insurance. Ensure you have enough cash reserves to survive this period if you choose to accept insurance and have few private-pay clients. Since the introduction of electronic billing and payments for providers, this has improved dramatically.

Challenges with Insurance Billing

Being in-network does not guarantee the insurance company will approve and pay your claims. Insurance companies use various tactics to delay or prevent payments. Often, clinicians receive denials for reasons like "failing to provide a taxpayer ID number" on a superbill, even though the taxpayer ID number is pre-printed on every superbill. This necessitates resubmitting the superbill, delaying payment by another month. Your contract also strictly limits how you can work with a member of the insurance company's plan. If a client wants to pay out-of-pocket but is a member of that insurance plan, you cannot accept an out-of-pocket payment from them, only their co-pay.

Out-of-Network Billing

A popular method of allowing clients to use their insurance while receiving your full fee is OON billing. You charge your full fee for each session, and either the client, you, or an insurance billing company submits an OON claim to the insurance company on the client's behalf. The insurance company then processes the claim and reimburses the client based on their plan benefits. This type of billing works only for clients with Preferred Provider Organization (PPO) insurance policies. Clients with Health Maintenance Organization (HMO) or Exclusive Provider Organization (EPO) plans do not receive reimbursement for services provided outside of their network.

Insurance Billing Companies

Insurance billing companies handle benefit verifications, billing, denials, appeals, and communicate with your clients regarding insurance-related issues for a fee. They usually charge a setup fee when you initially contract with them and then a percentage of the amount you bill each month. Setup fees average around $300, and billing companies typically charge 7% to 10% of your total monthly claims.

National Provider Identifier (NPI) Number

If anyone submits a claim to insurance for your services, you will need a National Provider Identifier (NPI) number. According to CMS.gov:

The National Provider Identifier (NPI) is a Health Insurance Portability and Accountability Act (HIPAA) Administrative Simplification Standard. The NPI is a unique identification number for covered healthcare providers. Covered healthcare providers and all health plans and healthcare clearinghouses must use the NPIs in the administrative and financial transactions adopted under HIPAA. The

NPI is a 10-position, intelligence-free numeric identifier (10-digit number). This means the numbers do not carry other information about healthcare providers, such as the state in which they live or their medical specialty.

If addiction counselors plan to bill insurance, they must register for an NPI number as covered healthcare providers. You can get your free NPI number immediately at the National Plan and Provider Enumeration System (NPPES) website.

Chapter Nine

Your Complete Startup Plan

D oes the term "business plan" terrify you? You're not alone! But here's the good news: you don't have to write a business plan from scratch. This book is your business plan and I've already written it for you! In this chapter, we'll walk through the essentials you need to have in place to launch your practice. Although the list might seem long, I've helped counselors set up and launch their practices in less than a week. You can work at your own pace, but I suggest following the order laid out here. Each item builds on the previous one, providing a solid foundation for your practice.

Here are the essentials for your new business:

1. Office Space

2. Phone Number

3. Legal Structure

4. Domain Name

5. Email Address

6. Malpractice and General Liability Insurance

7. Professional Headshot

8. Website

9. Directory Profiles

10. Business Cards

11. Client Forms

12. Electronic Health Records (EHR) System

13. Business License

14. Bank Account(s)

15. Payment Processing

With these in place, your practice will be up and running! Once it's set up, we'll expand your marketing and streamline your processes. For now, focus on completing each item. Avoid overthinking; set them up as instructed. You can adjust or fine-tune most items later.

Legal Structure

There are three common legal structures for counselors: sole proprietor, limited liability company (LLC), or corporation (INC or CORP). In many states, there's also a Professional Corporation (PC) designed for healthcare professionals, although SUD counselors in California are currently ineligible. The major benefit of an LLC or corporation is protecting your personal assets from lawsuits. The downside of an LLC or corporation is that it adds tax complexity and requires annual fees. In California, LLCs and corporations must pay an annual franchise tax of $800. You might need both business and personal tax returns, often doubling tax preparation costs. An accountant is essential if you have an LLC or corporation.

If you have any personal assets, such as a home, savings, or retirement accounts, consider an LLC or corporation. Otherwise, start as a sole proprietor and form an LLC or corporation as your income and assets grow. Malpractice insurance typically covers losses up to your policy limit, usually $1,000,000/$3,000,000 or higher if you choose maximum coverage. I began as a sole proprietor and switched to a corporation as my assets increased.

For a sole proprietor, you need nothing more unless you use a name other than your own for your practice. For example, I can use my name "Michael O'Brien, CADC II, NCAC I," for the name of my private practice. If I prefer to use "Sunshine Addiction Counseling," I need to file a fictitious business name (FBN) or "Doing Business As" (DBA) permit with my local county. An FBN or DBA allows you to use a business name other than your own name without forming an LLC or corporation. The cost is approximately $60, depending on location.

For an LLC or corporation, secure the proper forms from your Secretary of State, complete and submit them. You need a certified copy of your articles of incorporation to open a bank account or credit card processing account under your business name. You'll need the corporation active to sign leases or other legal agreements. Filing an LLC or corporation takes two to six weeks, but many states offer expedited options.

Office Space

An office that is easily accessible, quiet, safe, and private is crucial. Never see clients in your home because of potential negative consequences. "Neutral ground" is the most ethical and safe option.

Key considerations for selecting an office:

- Accessibility for disabled persons

- Waiting area or lobby

- Client-accessible bathroom

- Adequate free parking

- Professional furnishings

- Strong cellular signal

It is important for your office to be accessible to disabled persons. Occasionally, a client may use a wheelchair or struggle with stairs. If they can't get into your office, it creates an uncomfortable scenario. Occasionally, a client may show up under the influence or impaired. The less they need to navigate, the safer it is.

A lobby for clients to wait in with access to a restroom is ideal. Clients waiting outside or in a hallway will likely feel uncomfortable, risking confidentiality issues. A lobby with a white noise device or light music will mask conversations in your office. A private restroom cleaned by a janitorial service is optimal. Shared restrooms are acceptable; keep a key in your lobby if it's locked. Always have extra keys, as they will inevitably get lost or go home with clients.

Ensure adequate free parking for yourself and clients. Avoid locations with no parking or paid parking. Ideally, your office is centrally located, near mass transit, and easily accessible from major freeways. Think of your county and surrounding counties as your geographical service area and choose a convenient, high-population-density location.

Don't overthink furnishings, artwork, décor, or refreshments. In my first year, I sublet a tiny office with grey walls, no art, no windows, and standard office chairs. I never offered clients water, coffee, or tea. The office was safe, clean, private, and easily accessible. My success was because of my ability to help people, not the office appearance. Spend minimally to create a safe, clean, comfortable environment, adding luxuries as revenue increases. Clients rarely complain about the lack of refreshments or décor.

For administrative tasks like faxing, printing, and copying, keep it simple. My office is solely for seeing clients and counseling. I handle administrative work from home, responding to voicemails, emails, and client inquiries in the morning. Then, I head to the office to see clients. I keep a folder with hard copies of releases of information, credit card authorization forms, extra client paperwork, and referral sheets, which I'll discuss later.

A strong cellular signal is crucial for making phone calls and emergencies. If the office has no signal and there's a medical emergency, it's a problem. It also ensures internet access from your phone if needed. Check your phone's signal when touring potential offices.

Subleasing part-time from an established professional or in a suite with multiple offices and clinicians is an excellent initial solution. Being located with other practitioners for referrals, consultations, and mutual support is highly beneficial. Subleasing is cost-effective for part-time work, allowing you to add days and expenses as your practice grows. Typically, subleases don't require long-term commitments, hefty deposits, or credit checks.

To find subleasing opportunities, visit Craigslist and select the proper geographic area. Under "Housing," click "Office/Commercial" and search for "therapist" or "counseling." Rates vary by location; subleasing an office every Tuesday in Los Angeles might cost $150/month, while in rural Idaho, it might be $50/month.

Alternative options include contacting other clinicians in private practice or using executive offices from companies like Regus or We-Work. Reach out to listing creators, meet to tour the office, and ensure it feels like a good fit. Revisit the office at night to check for adequate lighting and safety. If it feels unsafe, find another location.

Substance abuse clients are not more challenging or disruptive than standard mental health clients. Unfortunately, you may encounter mental health professionals subletting office space who hold biases against substance abuse clients. My clients have never caused problems in the lobby or committed crimes at the office. I've shared space with psychiatrists whose clients occasionally disturbed others, but mine never have. If you share an office with a psychiatrist, and one of their clients creates a disturbance, educating clients about the psychiatrist's work fosters understanding and compassion without interfering with their counseling.

You probably won't work from the same office forever. As your practice grows, you can move to larger or more suitable spaces. I moved offices four times in three years, each time to a larger space. Eventually, I leased an entire suite and began subletting to other clinicians. Moving is okay if it benefits you and your clients.

At some point, subleasing may become costlier than leasing your own office. Leasing your office allows subleasing to other professionals, reducing your expenses. Leasing commercial office space is more involved, often requiring multi-year leases, utility costs, hefty deposits, and credit checks. Ending commercial leases early can be costly. A commercial real estate broker can help secure suitable office space within your budget and negotiate on your behalf.

One caution: avoid "Fee Splitting," where you pay a portion of your hourly rate to the clinician you're subleasing from for each client, instead of a flat monthly rate. It creates accounting headaches and potential ethical issues if you receive referrals from that clinician. Stick with a flat monthly rate and avoid signing non-compete agreements in subleasing contracts.

White noise or sound masking is essential for maintaining confidentiality. Place devices outside your counseling office, in the lobby, to mask conversations. Options include a fountain, white noise machine, fan, or music. To ensure discussions are confidential, ask a friend to take a phone call in your office while you sit in the lobby. If you can hear them, your clients will hear your sessions in the lobby.

Finding and securing office space is time intensive and feels permanent because of the contract. It's crucial to secure office space first; without it, you can't practice. For malpractice insurance, website, client forms, business cards, business license, and more, you require an office address. It should be your first step.

Phone Number

The simplest and most cost-effective solution for your practice's phone number and voicemail is to set up a free Google Voice account. While it might be tempting to use your personal cellphone number, I highly recommend against it. Keeping your personal number confidential for friends, family, and private business helps maintain a clear boundary between your personal and professional life. Having a separate Google Voice account provides a clean record of all calls, voicemails, text messages, and outbound calls made for your practice. This separation is crucial if you ever need to produce phone records for legal purposes, ensuring your personal calls are not mixed with business calls.

A Google Voice account works just like a regular phone line. You'll receive a local telephone number in your area code, allowing you to receive calls, voicemails, and text messages. You can also record a personalized greeting for your private practice and change it as needed. When you receive a voicemail, Google will transcribe it and send you an email so you can read the message without listening to it. You can install the Google Voice application on your smartphone, which allows you to answer calls, listen to voicemail, and send text messages in real time. Outbound calls made from the app will display your new practice number instead of your personal mobile number. We will cover what to include in your voicemail message later in the book.

Domain Name

A domain name is your website's address, leading clients to the same location each time it's typed into a browser. It serves several essential functions for your practice. A good domain name should be easy for clients to remember and revisit. It also plays a crucial role in how search engines view and rank your website in search results. Your domain name will also be part of your email address.

Choose a domain name that is as short as possible and contains keywords potential clients might use when searching for services. For example, people looking for help with substance abuse issues might search for terms like "Addiction treatment near me" or "Alcohol Rehab Dayton Ohio." Search engines prioritize domain names with these keywords. Use terms like addiction, substance abuse, recovery, help, counseling, and combining them with a location is optimal.

Avoid words that might confuse search engines about your service category. I used to prefer the word addiction versus recovery in domain names because recovery can apply to many things other than substance abuse. However, recovery and substance use disorder are now the more accepted terms and are totally appropriate for a practice domain name.

For example, my website domain name is www.obrienaddictio n.com. It's simple, short, and includes my last name and the word addiction. Coupled with my site's content discussing my substance abuse services, this makes it easy for search engines to index and serve my site to people seeking help. For a practice in Arlington, Virginia, run by someone named David Smith, good domain name suggestions include:

ArlingtonAddictionServices.com

AddictionServicesArlington.com

ArlingtonAddictionHelp.com

DavidSmithAddictionRecovery.com

ArlingtonSubstanceAbuse.com

ArlingtonDrugAlcoholHelp.com

AddictionHelpArlington.com

ArlingtonAddictionCounselor.com

To check if a domain name is available, use an internet services provider like GoDaddy, which I've used for over a decade. They offer competitive prices, excellent support, and seamless integration of all necessary internet products.

Email Address

Your email address should be an extension of your domain name. If your domain is www.arlingtonaddictioncounselor.com, your email address could be mike@arlingtonaddictioncounselor.com. For a small additional monthly fee, you can add an email account to your domain name account. Avoid using personal or free email accounts like addictioncounselor@gmail.com, as they look less professional. A custom email address adds credibility and professionalism to your practice. Your first name and domain name make for a perfect email address.

Malpractice and General Liability Insurance

General liability insurance covers injuries that occur at your practice, damage to a visitor's property, or other issues like advertising injury, copyright violations, or cyberattack data intrusions. Professional liability, or "malpractice" insurance, covers clinical issues like inaccurate advice, misrepresentation, negligence, or other clinical problems. Insurance providers typically offer both in one annual policy. This insurance protects you and your assets from the full cost of defending against claims or damages awarded in a lawsuit. **You cannot practice without it.**

In my twelve years as an addiction counselor, no one has ever sued me for malpractice or a general liability issue. Running your practice professionally and ethically minimizes the risk of lawsuits. Addiction counselors are defendants in only 7% of malpractice lawsuits brought against the disciplines covered by my insurance provider, HPSO. Despite the low risk, lawsuits happen, so you should protect yourself. Your insurance company will hire an attorney for you and cover the cost if you are sued for any reason.

Most insurance companies offer coverage levels of $1,000,000/$3,000,000, meaning they cover up to $1 million per incident and up to $3 million total for multiple incidents. My new policy has a $3,000,000/$7,000,000 option for higher liability limits, which I recommend. I pay $165 per year for my policy. You can't retroactively increase your limits when sued, so the extra cost is worth the extra coverage and peace of mind.

Insurance policies remain in force for the period paid, covering you for incidents that occurred during the policy period. If you retire and are subsequently sued for an incident that occurred a year before retirement, the insurance company has a responsibility to defend you. Confirm that your policy provides lifelong coverage for the period you paid premiums.

More expensive policies do not always offer better protection or service. My carrier, HPSO, provides excellent coverage, customer service, and training on liability issues. They are also one of the most affordable options. You can find insurance providers through local certifying or licensing organizations and professional addiction associations.

Professional Headshot

A professional headshot is a critical marketing tool. It's the first impression clients have of you, helping them decide if you seem trustworthy, friendly, and professional. Research shows online personal ads with pictures receive approximately 70% more responses. Similarly, clients often skip counselors without photos and chose one who has a photo.

Your professional headshot should not convey sex appeal or look like a dating profile picture. Aim for a neat, professional, friendly, and happy appearance. Business casual attire is essential; looking too formal might make clients feel uncomfortable or underdressed. I've never worn a tie in private practice for this reason.

Professional photographers and studios typically charge $50 to $350 for headshots. I invested more in this area because you get what you pay for. Alternatively, a friend or family member can take a picture using a modern smartphone, which usually has a powerful enough camera. Many phones also have portrait settings and apps like Face-Tune to touch up photos. Natural settings, like a park, generate the best client responses.

Avoid selfies or outdated photos that don't reflect your current appearance. You don't want clients to be surprised when they meet you. Exclude animals, friends, or family members, and avoid personally identifiable backgrounds like your home. Browse the Psychology Today website to see professional headshots and emulate those you find appealing.

Important Update

Before diving into website content and creating text for an online profile, I want to inform readers of significant changes since the initial publication of this book. While I have kept sections explaining essential content for your website and online profiles, I recognize that this has been a stumbling block for many counselors. Creating a website or online profile can be a source of anxiety for most professionals trying to launch their private practice.

Fortunately, there's good news! At AddictionPrivatePractice.com, we have developed automated AI-based tools to handle these challenging tasks for you. By answering a few basic questions, our new tool will generate the content for your website and online profiles effortlessly. Visit our website for more information. You'll be amazed at how our tools will create high-quality content for you and how much it will impact your new client acquisition.

Website

Your website is your new business card, brochure, and television commercial all in one. Almost every client and professional you work with will visit it. You don't need an expensive, professionally designed site. A basic, clean website that educates clients about your services and helps them connect with you is sufficient.

When I started my practice, I overbuilt my website with too much information, which confused and dissuaded clients. Your website should not look like a treatment program; clients seeking private practice usually aren't seeking a program. Clients visiting your site want to know if you can help them, understand them, accept them, if your services are affordable, and how to contact you. Four simple pages are all you need:

- Home Page

- My Experience Page

- My Services Page

- My Fees Page

Now that AI is available to everyone, creating text for your new website or a profile description has never been easier. In fact, it has never been easier to create a website because all the major web hosting companies now offer AI website builders. I have created articles and training courses on AddictionprivatePractice.com that will show you how to use these tools for your private practice.

Home Page

Your home page is the first page visitors see. It should welcome clients and communicate understanding and empathy. Clearly state your contact information at the top and bottom of the page. Avoid dark or depressing themes and images. Clients want to feel hope and envision their lives improving. Include:

- A simple title or catchphrase

- Two or three paragraphs of text

- A menu linking to other pages

- Contact information

- A crisis disclaimer

The crisis disclaimer provides immediate help for distressed visitors and informs them you don't provide emergency services. It should read:

"If you are in crisis, call the National Suicide Prevention Lifeline, a free, 24-hour hotline, at 988 or (800) 273-8255. If your issue is an emergency, call 911 or go to the nearest emergency room. I do not provide emergency services or immediate crisis support."

Write your text in a Word document or on paper to edit and revise as needed. Making an emotional connection is crucial.

My Experience Page

This page explains your qualifications without overdoing it. Use the title "My Experience" instead of "About Me" for a more professional feel. Include your professional headshot, a summary of your education, work experience, accomplishments, and professional memberships. Begin with a statement about the privilege of working with people who have substance abuse problems to balance the data about yourself.

Avoid presenting yourself as more important than your clients. List only relevant education and work experience. If you've written a book, created a program, or teach classes, include that. Keep personal life details private; clients may not choose you based on irrelevant personal preferences.

My Services Page

Outline and describe your services and the client process. Provide a one-paragraph description of each service and how it helps clients. Avoid overwhelming or confusing clients with too much information. Write from the heart to help clients connect with you. Remember, often less is better with websites - keep it simple!

My Fees Page

Clearly state your costs, financial policies, and insurance policies. Clients need fee information to make informed decisions. Without it, you'll get calls from clients who can't afford your services, wasting their time and yours. Outline what you charge for each service and provide links to free or low-cost services if needed.

Clients have to cancel or reschedule sessions 48 hours in advance to avoid being charged the full session fee. Make exceptions for documented emergencies. This boundary ensures the financial viability of your practice and supports clients' accountability. If you don't accept insurance, state that and offer a superbill for clients to submit for reimbursement. If you work with insurance, list the companies you're in-network with and explain how you handle benefits, authorization and deductible requirements. Specify your accepted payment forms.

Final Review and Publishing Your Site Live

After creating these pages, ask a colleague to review it for ethical and scope-of-practice issues. Once updated, publish your site. Your prospective clients understand you're a counselor, not a web designer. A clean, professional, caring website is all you need.

Business Cards

Despite the digital age, business cards remain relevant. A simple and plain design will do and is inexpensive. Include:

- Your name and credentials

- Address and phone number

- Website and email address

I add bullet points with my services, social media accounts, and a space for the client's next appointment time on the back. However, the essential items are enough. My basic black-and-white cards are effective, and my practice thrives. I've never had a client choose me because of a fantastic business card. They choose me because they believe they will get the help they need.

I create and order my cards through VistaPrint.com, choosing a professional design and customizing it with my information. They ship quickly, even with standard shipping. Keep it simple: select "Standard Business Cards," choose a design, and fill in your information. It's that easy.

> *Please note, the following forms are available on Addi ctionPrivatePractice.com.*

Client Forms

Client forms are the essential legal paperwork that clients must complete and sign before you provide services. Without these documents, you expose yourself to significant liability. Sometimes, state law requires that you provide your clients with a copy of these documents after they have signed them. Your client paperwork should include:

- Demographic Information and Intake Questionnaire

- The Informed Consent Document

- The Privacy Practices Notice (HIPAA)

- The Financial Agreement

- Payment Authorization Form

- Emergency Contact Release Form

- Telehealth Consent Form

Intake Questionnaire

The intake questionnaire consists of two parts. The first part collects the client's demographic information, including:

- Contact information (address, phone number, email address)

- Employment information

- Emergency contact information

- Date of birth, marital status, gender, sexual orientation, race, and religious affiliation

The second part collects necessary screening data in the client's own words. Clients should answer questions such as:

- Please describe the problem you need help with.

- What would you like to accomplish in counseling?

- Have you previously received counseling, therapy, or drug and alcohol treatment?

- What medications are you currently taking or have previously taken?

- Have you ever been hospitalized?

- Do you have any current medical conditions or are under a doctor's care?

- Are you currently feeling suicidal or homicidal?

- How is your relationship with your mother, father, and significant other?

- Does anyone in your immediate family have a history of substance abuse?

- Does anyone in your immediate family have a history of mental health issues?

- Have you ever been arrested for any reason?

- Are you currently being sued or suing anyone?

- Which substances do you currently use?

- Describe any significant trauma you have experienced in the last two years.

These questions are crucial as they help determine if the client is appropriate for your services and protect you legally. They also highlight whether a client might need a higher level of care or further investigation during the assessment. We will discuss handling these situations later, but for now, ensure your intake questionnaire is comprehensive and covers all relevant areas.

Informed Consent

The informed consent is a legal document that outlines the relationship between you and the client, detailing each party's responsibilities and providing essential information. This form should include:

- Your credentials, scope of practice, and education

- Your contact information, instructions on how to reach you after hours, and expected response times

- Common negative emotions and feelings clients may experience during counseling or recovery

- Issues that counselors are mandated to report and under what circumstances

- How missed appointments or late cancellations are handled

- Basic information on confidentiality

- What to do in emergencies

- How you handle impaired clients

- The transfer plan if your practice suddenly closes due to unexpected death or disability

- Your social media protocols and how you handle encounters with clients in public

- Coordination of care with other clinicians the client may be working with

Failing to inform your client of the above information does not allow them to give proper consent and may constitute malpractice. I review this document with clients in the first session to ensure they understand everything correctly.

Notice of Privacy Practices

The Notice of Privacy Practices includes information on both HIPAA and CFR 42 as it relates to substance abuse counseling. You must fully understand and explain these to your clients. Besides the Notice of Privacy Practices, I provide a basic synopsis of mandated reporting requirements in my client welcome email and verbally state the following for clients in our initial meeting, documenting it in my session notes:

"Everything you say in your assessment or counseling session is completely confidential and protected by law, with a few exceptions. I am mandated by law to report if you plan to harm yourself or someone else or if you report abuse of an elderly person, disabled person, or child. There are also certain circumstances where I might need to disclose information, detailed in the privacy notice you signed with your initial client paperwork. Please read it carefully. Do you have any questions regarding this information?"

This routine ensures that clients understand their privacy rights, and I always document it in my session notes.

Financial Agreement

The financial agreement is a separate document from the informed consent. It should clearly outline:

- Your fees for various services and accepted payment forms

- Your insurance billing policy

- How and when you collect payments and provide receipts

- What happens if a client fails to pay

- Your policy on late cancellations or rescheduling of appointments and the associated fees

These policies are crucial for avoiding misunderstandings and maintaining clear boundaries with clients.

Payment Authorization Form

I recommend accepting credit cards for payment. Most clients carry debit or credit cards, simplifying payment and accounting. If you accept credit cards, you need to keep a payment authorization form in the client's file. The form should include:

- A statement of authorization to charge the client's card

- The client's card information

- The client's address

- The client's signature

Maintain all intake forms in various formats (Word, PDF, hard copies) to accommodate different scenarios. Electronic Health Records (EHR) systems can streamline this process, allowing clients to review, complete, and sign forms electronically before their appointment.

Creating these documents from scratch is time-consuming and can result in missing critical information. Instead, download the forms provided through my website, enter your specific information, and your forms will be ready. I update these forms regularly to comply with changing laws and regulations, ensuring you always have the most current versions.

Electronic Health Records (EHR) System

Throughout my career, I have used various EHR systems. I recommend using an electronic system for 24/7 access to client files and schedules. An EHR system can help you:

- Digitally deliver new client paperwork and enroll new clients

- Maintain proper client documentation, including forms, releases, assessment information, progress notes, drug test results, and more

- Schedule clients and manage your weekly calendar

- Automatically send appointment reminders by text message or email

The EHR system I recommend for addiction private practices is SimplePractice, which offers:

- Affordable monthly pricing based on the number of clients

- Integrated Wiley Practice Planners for pre-written counseling goals, objectives, and progress notes

- Customizable client scheduling and reminders

- A client portal for electronic paperwork, appointment management, and billing

- Clinical supervision features

- Secure messaging that conforms to HIPAA compliance standards

- Excellent customer support and a free three-week trial

With SimplePractice in place, you'll be ready to move on to the next steps in opening your practice.

Business License

Almost all cities or counties require a business license to conduct business as a counselor. You can usually complete this online. If your office is in an unincorporated part of a county, check the county services website for requirements. Typically, authorities grant business licenses automatically upon payment of fees and they renew annually.

Please know that most cities now have code enforcement officers that go around the city and check for any violations. They go into commercial buildings and check each business to make sure they have their business license posted. Businesses that do not have a business license often face a stiff fine.

Bank Accounts

Having separate bank accounts for your practice simplifies accounting. Whether you are a sole proprietor or an LLC/corporation, you should have:

- Checking account

- Savings account for taxes

- Savings account for reserve funds

For corporate accounts, bring the following to the bank when you open an account:

- Government-issued ID

- Certified copy of your LLC or corporation articles of incorporation

- Business license

- Banking resolution (a document stating you may open bank

accounts for the corporation)

You will find a sample copy of a banking resolution at Addiction PrivatePractice.com

Payment Processing

Accepting credit cards as payment for your services is essential. To do this, you need a merchant account, which allows you to charge credit cards and deposit those funds into your chosen bank account. There are many companies where you can establish a merchant account, but I have found one I prefer and have used for many years—Square, Inc.

Square Inc. is a popular provider of merchant account services for millions of small businesses across the country. They offer a full range of small business services in addition to credit card processing. One of the most significant advantages of using Square is the ability to receive your funds instantly. While most merchant accounts take three to ten days to deposit funds into your bank account, Square allows you to deposit funds received from client credit card charges instantly.

This feature can be beneficial when you are just starting your practice and have not yet established a steady income. Square's fees are comparable to those of most major banks and merchant accounts. The setup process is straightforward—you only need to fill out one form, and you can start charging credit cards the same day. Unlike other merchant accounts, which often require multiple applications for American Express, Discover, and other smaller card issuers, Square streamlines this process.

What is the downside to using Square as your merchant account? In my experience, there isn't one. Square offers a reliable, efficient, and user-friendly solution for credit card processing, making it an excellent choice for your practice.

Chapter Ten

Marketing Essentials

Let's imagine for a moment that you're a working professional who feels like your drinking has become problematic. You
don't have withdrawal symptoms, legal issues, or work or relationship
problems because of your drinking, but you'd like to discuss your
concerns and make some changes before things get out of control. You
simply want to understand your problem better and start taking steps
to address it. You would think that for someone in this position, it
would be easy to find help. You search on Google, Bing, or Yahoo and
find therapist directories and a multitude of treatment programs. You
call several psychologists and therapists who either never return your
call or don't help people with addiction issues. While your problem is
concerning, you're sure you don't need a thirty-day addiction treatment program to get it under control—you're stuck.

There are millions of people across the United States in this same
predicament, and they often become so discouraged that they stop
looking for help. Then their problem eventually escalates to where

they actually need a higher level of care to resolve it. The system is broken and riddled with barriers to entry.

Believe it or not, despite the success of my practice over the years, marketing *isn't* something I spend much time or money on. This is shocking to most counselors, especially those who have invested heavily in marketing but still struggle with low-volume practices. You can duplicate my success by conducting the marketing activities described in this chapter. Most counselors who execute these marketing strategies will find they acquire new clients almost immediately.

As addiction counselors, we have some unique advantages over other types of mental health professionals. If you search the various online therapist directories, there are very few counselors in private practice who specialize in addiction. In many areas, there are no addiction counselors at all. There are, however, many mental health professionals who treat every issue a person could have. Clinicians who treat everything struggle to maintain a decent client load. One trend in mental health marketing over the past few years has been "niche" marketing, or focusing on a specialty area of therapy and targeting those specific clients. As an addiction counselor, you already have a niche, and it is one that is in high demand.

While psychologists, LMFTs, and LPCCs get some training and education on substance abuse issues, the vast majority focus on other mental health issues. Many of those clinicians even refuse to work with clients with addiction issues. Clients are looking for people who specialize in their specific issues and are effective at helping them resolve these issues. If you have cancer, you don't go to your family physician, who is a general practitioner. You go to an oncologist. Most clients feel the same way about addiction. When they see someone who simply tells them to go to Alcoholics Anonymous, they become discouraged and quit. They are looking for the tools, strategies, and experience that addiction counselors can provide. We're going to make sure they can find you!

Here are the marketing activities you need to accomplish to acquire new clients:

- Create profiles in directories that help clients find counselors.

- Connect with Board Certified Addiction Physicians in your area.

- Connect with Criminal and Family Law Attorneys in your area.

- Connect with Psychiatrists, Psychologists, Therapists, and Counselors in your area.

- Tour and develop working relationships with local alcohol and drug treatment programs.

- Go to AddictionPrivatePractice.com and learn about the additional marketing strategies that work.

Psychology Today and Other Online Directories

Important Update - There are some marketing strategies that were simply too valuable to put in this book. Visit AddictionPrivatePractice.com and learn about my proprietary marketing strategy that any counselor can use and get new clients. It is a simple system that requires no networking, cold calling, or other anxiety producing activities - and it works! Psychology Today also frequent-

> *ly changes its interface. My website will have the most up-to-date directions on how to complete your profile.*

My number one source of referrals is online directories. If you are searching online for help, Google will serve up thousands of search results packed with treatment programs, directories, and every addiction website known to man. Where does everyone look first? One of the online directories. It's the first place people look when they don't want information on programs. If you aren't in the directories, no one will find you.

Initially, 99% of my new client referrals came from these directories. Many years later, approximately 80% of my new clients still come from online directories, and the other 20% are from all other referral sources. The largest online directory for mental health professionals is Psychology Today. *95% of my new client referrals from directories come from Psychology Today.* The rest of the directories are nearly insignificant to my business, but I do my best to be listed in as many as possible.

One additional benefit of listing in as many directories as possible is that they create backlinks to your website. A backlink is when another website links back to your website. The more backlinks you have from reputable websites, the higher your website will come up in search rankings on Google, Bing, and Yahoo. For now, just remember that the more links to your website, the better!

Psychology Today has millions of visitors each month, and they pay Google and other search engines to be listed as one of the first search results when someone types in a search like "family therapist Chicago" or "addiction counselor Portland." Before you build your profile, go to PsychologyToday.com, click on "Find A Therapist," enter your zip code, and click the blue magnifying glass. You'll now see a list of therapists, counselors, and psychologists in your zip code. Click on the link to the left that says "Addiction" under the Issues heading in the side menu. You'll see a list of every therapist, counselor, and psychologist who is paying to have a profile on Psychology Today and claims they treat addiction in that specific area. Chances are there will be a long list because so many practitioners check all the boxes available, thinking they can treat anything and everything. Prospective clients don't like that; they are looking for an addiction counselor, not a counselor who does everything. There will probably be few or no actual addiction counselors on the list; if not—that's good for you! If there is, that's OK too. As our ranks grow and more people enter private practice, you will have more competitors. It's a fact of life. Trust me when I say that there are more than enough people looking for help than there are available addiction counselors.

Now, let's get your profile up! With Psychology Today, you'll receive six free months of being listed in the directory for free! That's $180 in free advertising! If you think $30 is a lot to spend each month for a profile—I can assure you, it's not. Even if you only signed up one new client per month, it is worth it. You don't have to start from scratch and come up with completely new text for your profile. Use the profile builder tool at AddictionPrivatePractice.com to create compelling profile text in seconds. Since the amount of text allowed in your profile is limited, you should only use the best copy from your website. In addition, you can use up to three additional zip codes in your profile so that people in the surrounding areas can find you. Go ahead and get your profile started, and I will walk you through each area! I'll discuss each section of the creation of your profile as you move along.

Name and Address

This section is fairly straightforward, but I'll give you some additional tips. Be sure to enter your website address; this is the only place you need to enter it. Under Primary Location, enter your office address. I suggest you check the box that says "Hide this street address from public view." This will make your actual address confidential, but still list your profile in the correct area so people can find you. You will also see a section called *Additional Location*. Some clinicians work at different offices at certain times of the week, which is why this field exists. What people don't realize is that if you leave this space blank, you are making a very expensive mistake. This is one of the additional zip codes you can show up in when new potential clients are looking for you. If you don't have a second location, you're going to create an imaginary one, and I'll show you the best way to do that.

First, go to the **Profile Zip Code Tool** on AddictionPrivateP ractice.com and follow the instructions. Higher population = more potential clients, a simple but incredibly important equation. The more people that see your profile, the more clients you will have. This tool will help you identify those zip codes and use them in your profile. The tool will also help you identify a neutral address. This is the address you will enter in the "Additional Location" address field. Then check the box that says, "Hide this street address from public view." It's important that you check that box; you don't want prospective clients showing up at the neutral address by accident. This will hide the address but still allow your profile to come up in one of the most populated zip codes in your county. You can then put in the address you'd like your monthly physical copy of "Psychology Today" to arrive at. Don't forget to click the save button.

Nearby Areas

This next section has two spots for additional zip codes you would like your profile to show in. Use the two additional zip codes you wrote down. Add zip codes and then save your work. Now your profile will show in a total of four zip codes! It will dramatically increase your profile response rate by being in the most populated zip codes in your county. Most clinicians never think of this and do not add nearby areas or an additional location—it gives you an important strategic advantage over them. Don't get tempted to just list the other zip codes near you because they are close and most convenient for clients. You should be listed in the most populous zip codes in your county. You will also often automatically come up in the areas near the zip codes you have entered.

Credentials

Complete the credential information. List your most important degree and school, not every single one of them. List the year you started working as a counselor. I started counseling when I began my practicum work in college, so that is the year I use. List your certifications, licenses, and any associations of which you are a member.

Specialties

Before we conquer this section of your profile, I'd like you to proceed with caution regarding the next few areas of your profile. Many counselors check every box they can hoping to attract potential clients. This is a huge mistake and can be catastrophic for addiction counselors. Do not select items that are out of your scope of practice. Some counselors may think that checking the box for obesity could mean you help obese people with addiction issues—that is not the case. It is specifically for treating obesity. Before you check any specialty, issue, or modality, ask yourself whether this is within your scope of practice. Is this something you're trained to do and can legally counsel someone for? Are you certified or trained in using this technique? If the answer is no, don't check that box. You could lose your certification or license over it, and many people have had their certifications suspended or revoked.

For Top Specialty 1, select Addiction.

For 2, select Alcohol Abuse.

For 3, select Substance Abuse.

Selecting these ensures you will always come up under the Addiction link when people are searching and not under other areas that aren't within your scope of practice. Under Issues, you can check the boxes related to your scope of practice that you feel you can help people in areas such as Addiction, Alcohol Abuse, Chronic Relapse, Codependency, Coping Skills, Drug Abuse, and Substance Abuse. I stick to areas pertaining to substance abuse, not behavioral addictions like Internet addiction, sex, gambling, shopping, or food. If you have special training or certifications in those areas and are qualified to work with people who have them, by all means, check them! If not, leave them blank. Leave all the boxes under Mental Health blank and the boxes under Sexuality. You will have another area to show that you specialize in working with LGBTQ clients; this area is specifically for working with clients who need help in those areas but aren't necessarily chemically dependent. Under "Other Issues," I like manually add "DUI & Court Mandated Counseling or Evaluations" and "Alcohol & Drug Assessments" as many prospective clients search on those terms when looking for help and need those services. It also adds some more valuable keywords to your profile when search engines index it. You may also list other services you offer, like interventions or consultations. Save your work and move to the next section.

Treatment Preferences

This can be another slippery area with the scope of practice. While I'm aware of and have had some education on cognitive behavioral therapy (CBT), dialectical behavioral therapy (DBT), person-centered therapy, and positive psychology, I do not check those boxes. These boxes indicate what treatment a potential client prefers. I stick with coaching and motivational interviewing because they are the only treatment preferences that apply to me and are not out of my scope of practice. Then under "Other Treatment Orientation," I list "12-Step & Non-12-Step Counseling" and "Drug Testing Available". You may also add substance abuse counseling, drug abuse counseling, or chemical dependency counseling. Under modality, I only choose "Individuals". You may also check "Group Counseling" if you plan to offer groups to your clients.

Client Focus

Under "Age Specialty," I only specify *Adults* and *Elders* as those are the two age groups I work with. Under Religious Orientation, I select "*Any*." I choose no other special categories or ethnicities, and I don't speak any other languages, but if you do and are fluent enough to counsel in that language, you can list it. If you have any special insight or training in working with the special populations listed, check them. If you speak another language fluently enough to conduct counseling, you can market specifically to members of that ethnic group in many ways. Non–English-speaking communities are woefully underserved

all across the United States, and we more bilingual addiction specialists.

Finances

Your session cost range should be the cost of the lowest and the highest
of your services. I do not offer initial free face-to-face consultations
because they can be very time-consuming and my schedule is too busy,
but I offer free phone consultations of 30 minutes or less to potential
clients. Please note that if your practice is full to the point, you can't
take on any new clients, you have the option to show that in your
profile. Select the forms of payment you accept. I suggest you avoid
PayPal; their policies can make disagreements with clients or even
just receiving your legitimate payments difficult, and it isn't worth
the hassle. If you do not accept insurance, select "No." Check the
Out-of-Network box as some clients may choose to submit superbills
from you and seek reimbursement from their insurance company.
List your malpractice insurance carrier information and leave the NPI
number blank.

Personal Statement

Other than your professional headshot, this is the most important
piece that prospective clients use when deciding about whether to use
your services. You can use the Profile Builder tool on AddictionPriv
atePractice.com for the perfect personal statement. Psychology Today
provides its own guidance for each section of the personal statement,
but I have found that a slightly modified approach to their content
suggestions works best for addiction counselors. Use paragraph one
to address how you understand addiction and what the prospective

client is going through. In paragraph two, be specific about what you offer that will help those addiction clients. In paragraph three, include a call to action like "Get your substance abuse assessment, call today!" If there is anything unique about the population you serve, or the type of services you offer, you may also state it here; otherwise, it will just be an extension of paragraph two with a call to action. Double-check your spelling and grammar.

The mistakes I commonly see counselors make here are that they fail to let the client know they understand them or explain how they can help them. They list things like the school they graduated from in their statement! The client doesn't care about that. They also list too many things that they do instead of a few core things that most clients need. Make an emotional connection and you'll be far ahead of your competition and get more new clients. Your potential clients want to know you understand what they are going through.

Don't forget to upload your professional headshot or photograph. Save your profile and then submit a copy of your certification or license to Psychology Today so that they can verify it. They will look you up and make sure your credential is valid, and then you'll receive the "Verified by Psychology Today" badge in the search results. You can use this information in other online profiles you create. The hard part is over.

Advanced Online Profile Marketing

For most clinicians, one profile will not provide a sufficient number of new clients to sustain their practice. I have developed a system for maximizing the power of Psychology Today and significantly boosting your new client calls in less than a week. Most counselors who employ my advanced marketing techniques don't need to do any additional marketing activities. You will be amazed at the results as the methods I teach you in this course build on the work you have done in your Psychology Today profile! Check it out if you would like to turbo charge your new client acquisition and reduce or eliminate the need for any other marketing. You will find this course on AddictionPriv atePractice.com.

Other Online Directories and Profiles

Now that you've done the work of creating your Psychology Today profile, you can use the same information for all of your other profiles in the other directories you choose to list yourself in. Here are some that I have found to be beneficial:

- Yelp
- Facing Addiction with NCADD
- SAMHSA–Behavioral Health Treatment Services Locator

Connect with Board-Certified Addiction Physicians

It wasn't long ago that finding a physician who was board certified in addiction medicine was nearly impossible. Thankfully, things have transformed over the last five years. More and more physicians are specializing in addiction medicine and going into private practice. While the American Society of Addiction Medicine (ASAM) has been around since 1954, it has really risen to prominence as the nation has grappled with the opioid epidemic.

Connecting and developing relationships with the addiction physicians in your area is critical to the success of your practice for two reasons: (1) you will need to refer clients for medical issues regularly, and (2) physicians don't provide counseling and will often provide a steady stream of referrals. I have sent hundreds of clients to see addiction physicians over the years, and I have received hundreds of referrals from them as well. My relationships with addiction physicians are some of my strongest ones, and several have become friends.

I guarantee you will have clients who need medical assistance when they stop using or drinking or need ongoing medical care after they stop. Emergency departments and urgent care clinics are good at handling life-or-death emergencies, and you will need to refer some clients there if they are having significant medical issues. Unfortunately, they are not very good at helping people with detox or other substance abuse-related medical issues. They do not provide any medication-assisted treatment. I have sent many clients to the emergency room with significant withdrawal symptoms only to have them turned away without so much as an aspirin. This is not only discouraging but dangerous for clients.

Addiction physicians in private practice can often evaluate and assist clients who need help with outpatient detoxification. In addition, they can provide ongoing medical and medication support for your clients in recovery. Some addiction physicians have counselors or therapists in their offices that do exactly what I do, but they almost always respect the referral relationship and do not poach my clients for their counselors.

Visit the ASAM website. Under the resources tab, you will see "Find a Doctor." Click that link and search for physicians in your area. I simply cold-called each doctor, and every single one of them called me back! They are always looking for good counseling resources for their clients. My initial voicemail to them would include something like the following:

Hi Dr. Smith, this is Michael O'Brien. I'm an addiction counselor and have recently launched a new private practice in your area. I'd really like to connect with you as I regularly have clients who need addiction medicine services. I'm hoping we can connect, as I'd love to pick up some of your business cards and learn more about your practice. My number is 555-555-5555 and my email is mike@sunshineaddictioncounseling.com. I look forward to hearing from you, thanks!

That's it! Short, sweet, and to the point. You never have to sell your practice. When you connect with them and find out more about their practice, they will ask you about yours. Be sure to bring your business cards when you visit them. Be sure to find out which insurance plans they accept, what their fees are, when they work, and what the best way to contact them is if you need to discuss a mutual client. You will need this information for clients when referring to them.

Connect with Criminal and Family Law Attorneys

Another symbiotic referral relationship is with criminal and family law attorneys. These two types of lawyers regularly have clients with substance abuse issues. They are also the attorneys that my clients most often seek services from. You will have clients with both criminal and family court matters who need legal representation.

An easy, fast way to make these connections is by searching Google using the term "Criminal attorney near me" or "Family law attorney near me." Start visiting the websites of the attorneys in your area and find their email address on their website. If you can't find an email address, a phone call will also work. Send out a minimum of five emails per day using this type of email:

Dear [Name],

Hello, my name is Michael O'Brien. I'm an addiction counselor and recently opened a private practice in [County]. I work with many clients who need legal services and rarely have legal representation. I am very interested in learning about your law practice and how you may best represent clients I may refer to you. I'd love to get to know you and establish a reciprocal referral relationship that benefits both of our clients. I am also making myself available to your clients who may need my services. I have twelve years of experience in the substance abuse treatment field working with a wide variety of clients from diverse backgrounds.

Through my private practice, I now provide substance abuse assessments and evaluations, aftercare (counseling for those who have completed residential treatment), counseling for individuals, drug testing, and consultations. I can provide counseling services for clients who are mandated by criminal or family courts as well as evaluations for most legal scenarios. As I am not affiliated with any treatment programs, I provide fair and objective assessments that truly meet the needs of the clients and provide effective recommendations.

May we schedule a brief introductory call or visit? I'd love to come by and pick up some of your business cards. Please send me any information you can provide on your practice. Thanks for your time.

Sincerely,

Michael O'Brien, CADC II, SAP, NCAC I

Website

Phone

Connect with Psychiatrists, Psychologists, Therapists, and Counselors in Your Area

While many clinicians see other clinicians as competition, I see them as strategic alliances that benefit my clients and my practice. As an addiction counselor, our scope of practice is very limited, and your clients will often need help from an additional professional. Most my clients have another disorder that compliments their substance abuse problem. The problems include but are not limited to ADHD, trauma, PTSD, depression, anxiety, and other issues. If a client can achieve sobriety and does not address these underlying issues, they will almost certainly relapse.

My clients frequently have what I refer to as an interdisciplinary team to help them achieve success. Here are some examples of how that may look in private practice:

- A married male client with children has been drinking heavily for years and has destroyed the trust he had with his family. The client is sober, but constantly triggered by the conflict with his wife and family. The entire family needs help recovering from alcohol abuse. In these situations, I refer my clients to one or more MFTs who can provide family therapy or therapy for the spouse and children. My client continues seeing me for substance abuse but simultaneously begins addressing their family problems once they have stabilized.

- A female client with ADHD and a history of sexual trauma had been smoking marijuana heavily and binge drinking. Here, I would refer my client to a psychiatrist for ADHD treatment and a therapist who specializes in trauma.

- A family brings in their college-age son who has become

alcohol dependent while away at college. I will often see the
student for alcohol dependency but refer him to an addiction
physician for help with his initial detox. While I may have one
or two educational sessions with the client and his family, I
always recommend that the parents see another professional
for their own support and give referrals.

When I initially started in private practice, I was concerned these
other types of professionals would see me as a subordinate. Nothing
could have been further from the truth. I have developed some powerful relationships with other providers, which have benefited hundreds
of our mutual clients. They treat me as a colleague and an equally
valuable professional. In fact, when I initially reached out to some
of these clinicians, I heard things like, "I am so glad you called! I've
been struggling to find professional addiction support for several of
my clients" or "I have a client whose drinking is really interfering with
his PTSD treatment." When you put a powerful team together that
truly addresses your client's problems, genuine change happens, and
the outcomes will astonish you.

Use Psychology Today to find clinicians in your area who specialize
in things other than addiction. Click through to their website from
their profile and find their email address. Do not send them an email
through Psychology Today. Psychology Today has spam filtering that
prevents such types of emails from getting through to the person you
are trying to reach. Once you have their actual email, send them a
customized email like this:

Dear [Name],

Hello, my name is Michael O'Brien. I'm an addiction counselor
and recently opened a private practice in [County]. Every so often, I

have clients who suffer from PTSD in addition to their addiction, and I see you specialize in treating PTSD on your website.

I work with many clients who need PTSD treatment, and I'm wondering if you would accept referrals from me? I am very interested in learning about your practice and how you help clients I refer to you. I would like to get to know you and establish a reciprocal referral relationship that benefits both of our clients. I am also making myself available to your clients who may need my services. I have twelve years of experience in the substance abuse treatment field working with a wide variety of clients from diverse backgrounds.

Through my private practice, I now provide substance abuse assessments and evaluations, aftercare (counseling for those who have completed residential treatment), counseling for individuals, drug testing, and consultations. As I am not affiliated with any treatment programs, I provide fair and objective assessments that truly meet the needs of the clients and provide effective recommendations.

May we schedule a brief introductory call or visit? I'd love to come by and pick up some of your business cards. Please send me any information you can provide on your practice. Thanks for your time.

Sincerely,

Michael O'Brien, CADC II, SAP, NCAC I

Website

Phone

Develop Relationships with Alcohol and Drug Treatment Programs

You will need to refer clients to higher levels of care from time to time. It is important to know the treatment programs in your area well and establish a relationship with them. There are two common scenarios in which I work with programs: (1) clients are referred to me for aftercare counseling after completing treatment, and (2) I determine that one of my clients requires a higher level of care, I refer that client to treatment, then resume counseling when they have completed their program.

Most programs do not offer one-on-one aftercare counseling on an ongoing basis to clients who have completed their program. Programs can include you in their client's aftercare plans or discharge instructions and will often call to set up the client's first appointment before they leave the facility. I reach out to the business development person at the program to schedule a tour, and I inform them I'd love to meet the clinical director, case managers, or others involved in discharge planning. I also pick up some of their marketing materials, so that I can provide them to clients who need referrals.

You will find that most programs will be very interested in developing a relationship with you. Here is a sample introductory email I send to programs:

Dear [Name],

Hello, my name is Michael O'Brien. I'm an addiction counselor and recently opened a private practice in [County]. I frequently refer clients to treatment, and I am interested in learning more about your program. Would you be able to provide me with a tour of your facility and marketing materials I may give to my clients? I am also very interested in meeting your clinical staff if possible.

Many clients who successfully complete treatment need ongoing aftercare counseling. I am happy to provide this to your clients and help improve their long-term outcomes. I have twelve years of experience in the substance abuse treatment field working with a wide variety of clients from diverse backgrounds. Through my private practice, I provide substance abuse assessments and evaluations, after-care (counseling for those who have completed residential treatment), counseling for individuals, drug testing, and consultations. As I am not affiliated with any other treatment programs, I can provide objective referrals to clients who would benefit from your program.

Thank you for your time, and I look forward to meeting you and touring your facility!

Sincerely,

Michael O'Brien, CADC II, SAP, NCAC I

Website

Phone

Notification and Acknowledgement of Referrals

Whenever I am referring clients to any other providers, once they have selected one, I ask them to sign a release of information so that I can coordinate care with the other provider. Clients usually appreciate this, as it sets them up for success and smooth intake with the other provider. Once I have a release, I will reach out to the other provider and let them know I made the referral and am happy to answer questions they have or provide background information. Any time I receive a referral from any other provider, I always send them a handwritten thank-you note. It's a personal touch that only takes thirty seconds but can have a lasting impact on your relationship with the provider. Find some Thank You cards on Amazon and keep them on hand with a supply of stamps.

Marketing Tactics to Avoid

There are many other ways to attract clients to your practice. The ones I have listed above are the most effective. However, you may develop other marketing methods that may help build your practice as well. Some counselors reach out to the student health offices at local colleges or universities, contact local physicians, join the chamber of commerce, or provide free informational classes for families or loved ones of someone with a substance abuse problem. Those are great ways to bring in more clients! There are a few marketing tactics, however, that should be avoided.

I have never given or received any type of compensation or incentives to/from other providers, clients, or programs for my practice to be successful. In California and many other states, it is now illegal to receive kickbacks or any other form of compensation for referrals. I have also seen clinicians of all disciplines use gimmicks—like offering a gift certificate to a restaurant for buying a certain number of sessions or some other type of shiny object—to attract clients. I have heard of counselors attending 12-step meetings and attempting to hand their cards or meet new potential clients. These types of marketing tactics seem desperate and, sometimes, may be an ethical violation or illegal.

I would also like to note that reciprocal referrals should not be required in order to refer to someone; in fact, it is unethical. While that is often the outcome when you find other clinicians who can help your clients, it should never be required. There are many situations in which I refer to another professional or program and have never received or never will receive a referral. I do it because it is the right thing to do for the client.

Chapter Eleven

Essential Consultant Relationships

N o private counselor can succeed alone. Developing critical consultant relationships right away is vital to ensure you avoid legal issues, financial mistakes, or malpractice lawsuits. Here are the key consultants you should have in place when starting your practice:

Accountant

Regardless of whether you are a sole proprietor, an LLC, or a corporation, you need an accountant. Properly withholding and paying taxes on time is crucial. Many clinicians make costly mistakes in their first few years by failing to do so. Depending on your legal structure, you may need to pay quarterly taxes or plan for large end-of-year tax bills. An accountant can help you decide on the most favorable legal structure for tax savings and tell you exactly how much to save for taxes from every fee you collect.

Setting up your tax and accounting processes from day one will save you time and money later. Each day I earn income, I allocate a percentage to my tax savings account, reserve savings account, and retirement fund. Developing this habit from day one is one of the smartest things you can do. Save receipts, monthly statements, credit card revenue reports, and track your expenses. I recommend FreshBooks, a top accounting program for small business owners, as it is user-friendly and cost-effective. Many online tax services like TurboTax or H&R Block offer consultations with tax professionals at reasonable prices. Many accountants also offer a free initial consultation. A skilled accountant can quickly answer important questions such as:

- What legal structure is most favorable for me financially?

- What percentage of my daily revenue should I withhold for taxes?

- What type of retirement account will save me the most on taxes?

Ask other counselors or professionals in private practice for recommendations. Call various accountants, inquire about their fees, and ask if they offer a free initial consultation.

Clinical Supervisor

If you're new to private practice, having a clinical supervisor is essential. They help you be the best counselor possible, protect your clients and yourself, and reduce potential liability. I recommend counselors new to private practice have clinical supervision for at least one year.

Your clinical supervisor should be a clinician with equal or higher credentials, who has been in private practice and has experience with substance use disorders.

Working in a team treatment environment usually provides built-in levels of accountability and supervision. You can recreate this security in private practice with a clinical supervisor, who helps you avoid mistakes and better serve your clients. I view clinical supervision as a coaching relationship designed to help me excel, not as a burden. Common mistakes new private practice counselors make without a clinical supervisor include:

- Wandering beyond their scope of practice

- Falling behind in charting or not doing it at all

- Failing to perform critical daily processes

- Not improving the quality and efficiency of their charting

- Violating ethics

Unexpected situations will arise in private practice where you need support or clinical consultation. Having someone to guide you through these scenarios is invaluable. Examples of such scenarios include:

- A client feeling suicidal

- A client disclosing a mandated reporting issue

- Providing an assessment report and recommendations to a court

- Developing romantic feelings for a client, or vice versa

- A client overdosing and being on life support

- A client's death

A clinical supervisor should at least:
  - Review new client intake paperwork

  - Review and approve your assessments, progress notes, and reports weekly

  - Provide feedback and coaching for areas of improvement

  - Offer clinical consultation and support

Emergency Coverage and Transition Counselor

Life is unpredictable, and it's crucial to have a plan for unexpected events. If you suddenly cannot practice because of an accident or unforeseen circumstances, an emergency coverage and transition counselor ensures your clients continue to receive care. This person should have the same or higher scope of practice and be legally able to provide services to your clients. Ideally, they should know you well enough to step in if needed. If not, a close family member or friend should know who to contact.

A trusted colleague and I provide this service to each other reciprocally at no cost. I include their name in my informed consent document, give them a key to my office, provide them with a code for the security system, share my voicemail password, and grant them access to my client files, contacts, and email. Your transfer plan should include:

- Notifying all active clients of your inability to practice

- Providing counseling or referral services to active clients

- Taking possession of all client clinical records and maintaining them for seven years

- Responding to all records requests as permitted under current confidentiality laws and regulations

- Destroying client clinical records after seven years

Both counselors should maintain a notarized original version of the agreement. Provide a copy to a close family member, your attorney, or with your will or estate information. While these duties may seem ominous, they are manageable. I've provided these services for colleagues and found it helped me cope with grief, giving me a strong sense of duty to their clients. While not seeking to profit from unfortunate circumstances, many clients may request that you become their counselor, providing some compensation for your efforts.

If you don't have a colleague who can provide these services, join our online community at AddictionPrivatePractice.com. You can connect with other counselors who can provide this service.

Chapter Twelve

Financial Management

Having a regular job has the advantage of including some critical financial management tasks right in your paycheck. When you receive a paycheck from an employer, they take out taxes, health insurance premiums, and retirement contributions, and you typically build up paid-time-off (PTO). This may result in you receiving half of your gross pay, but these critical obligations are covered, so you don't have to think much about them. In private practice, you are the one who has to do it. One of the biggest mistakes I see counselors make is that they don't pay attention to financial management and develop good practices starting on day one. If you don't put these practices into place right away, you will get used to living off your gross monthly income, and implementing them later is much tougher! It feels like your income goes down considerably. Don't let a crisis be what forces you to adopt responsible financial management habits.

With taxes, if you aren't saving for your expected tax liability, you will end up with a major tax bill at the end of the year that you can't pay. If you have a healthy practice and don't save for taxes, and your tax bill is $25,000, where would you come up with that money? What compounds this problem is that the state and IRS will add severe penalties and interest to whatever amount you owe. This means you could pay 25% or more in additional taxes that you didn't need to. Let's examine how I handle my financial management.

Federal and State Taxes

Let's assume that after your first year, you have a full client load and business is booming. In California, at $125 per hour, my income would be $160,000. That means my federal tax bracket would be 24%, the federal self-employment tax is an additional 15.30%, and my California tax bracket will be 9.30%. My total tax liability could be as high as 49% of my income. It actually never is 49%. After I receive my standard deductions, deduct health care premiums and costs, and all my business expenses, this number comes down dramatically. Usually, I pay closer to 35% of my total income in taxes: 35% of $160,000 is $56,000. That is the amount I should have paid in quarterly tax payments throughout the year. This figure may be different depending on your legal structure, and you should discuss these figures with your accountant, but for now, we will assume most people are sole proprietors.

In the start-up plan, one task was to set up a checking account and multiple savings accounts. One of those should be your tax savings account. Every day that I have revenue, I transfer 35% of it into my tax savings account. When my accountant tells me what my quarterly tax payment is, I then move the required amount to my checking account, write a check, and send it in. Since I have been dutifully saving 35% of my daily revenue, paying my taxes has been fairly pain free over the years. You must consult with a tax professional even if you use the worksheet I have created.

What happens if you save too much money for taxes? You get a bonus at the end of the year! I do my best to not save too much or too little, and it usually works out that I save too much. This is your money to do with as you please. I typically transfer any extra tax savings into my retirement account.

Benefits Cost and Savings

Another major expense for the self-employed is paying for your own benefits. When I first started my practice, I only bought a health insurance plan. As my practice grew and my income became very stable, I added more benefits that I could now afford. My current benefits include:

- Medical insurance

- Dental insurance

- Vision insurance

- Life insurance

- Disability insurance

- Long-term care insurance

Thanks to the Affordable Care Act, purchasing medical insurance has become much easier and less expensive for most people. If you leave your job to go into private practice and leave behind your benefits, that usually qualifies you to immediately sign up for benefits. The great thing about using a health exchange or Covered California or

Healthcare.gov is that you can start out with a realistic lower annual income, which may qualify you for lower premiums and subsidies to offset those premiums. As your income increases, you simply notify your insurance exchange, and your premiums may increase, and your subsidies will decrease, but you will be better able to afford them at that point.

Because of my income level, I receive no subsidies on my premiums, but they are tax deductible. You do not need to acquire all of these policies when you first start your practice. I recommend you start with medical insurance and add in the additional policies when your income can support them. My current costs for these policies are:

- Medical $485 per month

- Dental $32 per month

- Vision $24 per month

- Life $92 per month

- Disability $118 per month

- Long-Term Care $44 per month

Your total cost is $795 per month.

Policy costs can vary dramatically based on where you live, your age, and your health conditions. Two things are for sure: insurance never gets cheaper, and coverage becomes more expensive as you age. My annual insurance premiums are approximately 6% of my income. Every day that I have revenue, I put 6% into my reserve savings account. Do some research on what these policies will cost you and plug them into the financial management worksheet.

Paid Time Off (PTO) Savings

When you work for yourself and you can't work, you don't get paid. When I take vacations, I feel as if the cost is double in private practice. It's double because you don't receive any income on the days you are on vacation, and you still have to pay for the vacation! When you see clients in your office, they will bring in every germ possible. If you catch the flu and cannot counsel for three or four days, it can really affect your earnings for the month.

To prepare for sick days or vacations, I have a reserve savings account. At my income level, saving 5% of my daily revenue results in $8,000 in savings by the end of the year. That usually covers me for one or two days of illness and a nice vacation or two. You can start with a lower number in the beginning and increase it as your income becomes stronger.

Retirement Savings

I don't want to survive on Social Security when I retire. Some very basic planning and savings can make a vast difference in the quality of your retirement. Technology has made retirement savings and investment easier than it has ever been. For the longest time, I did my best to put away $500 per month toward retirement. Now that I'm getting older, I make sure I save at least $1,000 per month. These savings add up quickly! At some point, as I get closer to retirement, I may actually be able to reduce my savings as I have made great strides in achieving my goals. Saving $12,000 per year requires me to transfer 7.5% of my daily income into my retirement account.

There are thousands of options for saving for retirement. Too many, and if you aren't careful, you could waste a substantial amount of your retirement savings on fees for mutual funds and the accounts that hold them. Luckily, I have found one of the easiest and least expensive retirement accounts possible! In August 2014, Acorns was launched and quickly grew into a serious player in the retirement savings industry. Acorns offers innovative ways of saving for retirement that make companies like Fidelity or Schwab cringe.

The retirement investment options cost $1, $2, or $3 per month! Not per transaction or trade—per month! And the mutual or index funds they offer are no-fee or very low-fee. There are also multiple ways to boost your retirement savings. Of course, you can simply transfer money into your retirement account with their easy-to-use app. But they offer two more unique savings methods that have significantly boosted my savings over the years.

Acorns has also forged relationships with many of the brands and services you use every day. Acorns calls it *"Found Money."* Companies like AT&T, Walgreens, Wal-Mart, Airbnb, and Lyft will contribute either a lump sum to your retirement account for joining their service or a percentage of your purchase. Many of the companies you use every day take part, and the contributions to your retirement account on an annual level can be significant. It's like free retirement money for the things you already buy. They even have a web browser extension that alerts you any time you can grab some of this found money.

If you aren't using Acorns, you are probably paying too much for your retirement accounts and mutual funds, and you're leaving free money on the table. You will find a link to the correct Acorns on AddictionPrivatePractice.com. There are several companies out there with that name, so use the link to be sure you get to the right one.

Total Monthly Costs

We've gone over all of the various things you should save for on a monthly basis. What does the financial breakdown look like? Here is mine:

Monthly Revenue $13,300

Tax Savings (35%) $4,655

Insurance Premiums (7.5%) $997

PTO Savings (5%) $665

Retirement Savings $1,000

Total Monthly Deductions $6,317

Net Monthly Income $6,982

Yes, that is nearly 50% of my income. Some of it, like taxes, is unavoidable. With insurance, PTO, and retirement, you can start off slow and build as you go. That 50% buys me incredible peace of mind and covers me for every scenario. You will pay for health care one way or another; insurance is the best way to do it! You will get sick, you will need time off, and you will eventually have to retire. This is the financial blueprint for my success, safety, and security. I hope you implement these strategies right away and avoid learning these lessons the hard way.

Chapter Thirteen

Billing

You can't run a successful practice without billing. Done correctly, it can be painless for you and your clients. The system I have developed is foreign to most counselors, but when they learn it, they often quickly adopt it. Letting your billing get out of control can adversely affect you and your clients. If your clients experience this system from their first visit, they quickly get used to it. You almost never have to discuss payments, and you never have to use a collection agency. In fact, over the many years I have been in private practice, I have never once had a credit card charge disputed and I have received only one bounced check.

At the time of intake, I ask all of my clients to provide a credit or debit card and sign an authorization for me to charge it. I require them to keep this information up to date and send them a new form if their card information changes. I discourage using other types of payment by requiring that a deposit, equal to one session fee, must be retained if they choose to pay by cash or check. Why would I discourage cash or checks when there is no transaction fee for accepting them as payment? Because, over time, you will be unable to collect missed session fees in cash or payments for bounced checks. The small transaction fee for you to charge their card is worth saving a trip to the bank and the security of the payment. With my appointment reminders, financial agreement, and credit card authorization form, it would be nearly impossible for a client to dispute the charge, and it has never happened in my practice.

As my informed consent, financial agreement, and payment authorization form state, I charge all of my clients for their services on the morning of their scheduled service. As you will see in the daily operations flow chart, billing is the first thing I do every morning. Doing so prevents many problems, such as:

1. **Clients who have not canceled within 48 hours of their appointment must pay the full fee for their late-canceled or rescheduled session.** Therefore, I am owed that fee at the time that I charge my clients. If we were to compare how many no-shows, late cancellations, or late reschedules other counselors who do not use this system have and myself—I'm certain I have far fewer. If a client has paid for their session, they are much less likely to cancel or not show up because they have already paid, and they don't want to forfeit that payment. Clients are aware of this because of the documents they sign, and I also remind them in the welcome email and on our first visit.

2. **It saves time during sessions.** Every minute counts in a session. If you are dealing with payment and delivering a receipt in the session, you are wasting counseling time. This takes at least five minutes and can take longer if the client forgets their wallet in the car, forgets the payment altogether, has to write a check, or there is some technical issue with you issuing the receipt.

3. **It models healthy boundaries.** This system feels very professional to clients, and it models good boundaries. You are abiding by the terms of your agreement with the client and they should do the same. You are also showing your worth and the value of your services.

4. **It prevents most of the tough conversations.** Most substance abuse clients have issues with their finances or managing them. This system avoids having conversations with clients about forgetting payments, bouncing checks, or even the awkward collecting payment talk at the beginning or end of each session. If a client misses an appointment, then comes to their next session, you now have a double payment to collect. Preventative measures that make these conversations as rare as possible are good for your client and your relationship with them.

5. **It prevents you from not getting paid and your clients from having to pay extra fees.** If a client's card declines when I bill them in the morning, I reach out to them by email, phone, or text and let them know. This gives clients time to arrange for a new method of payment or to update their payment information. If a client cannot pay that day, I get to decide in advance how I would like to handle that. I have created a "*Session Fee Did Not Process*" email. Bounced checks also come with a price tag. Usually, you charge the client an additional fee for a bounced check, and so does their bank. This system eliminates extra fees.

6. **It keeps you focused on the clients and not on business while in sessions.** There is no better feeling than leaving for the office, having the money in the bank for the eight sessions I have that day, and never once having to discuss business with a client. However, if you are leaving for the office unsure about who will show up and bring their payments, distracted by conversations about payment, your day gets much more complicated. When a client arrives at my office, they have been charged for their session and have a receipt automatically delivered to their email.

I have never lost a client or failed to sign one up because of this billing system. I've had no chargebacks or complaints about my billing processes. It's clean and straightforward to the benefit of the client and myself. Now, let's look at the backend of billing. Here are the tasks I complete when I bill clients:

1. I charge their card using Square; they receive an automated receipt in an email.

2. I record their payment in SimplePractice.

3. If a client's card declines, I send them the "*Session Fee Did Not Process*" email and if there is no response before I leave for the office. I text them asking them to please check their email.

4. I transfer the payments from Square, to my business checking account.

5. If billing insurance, I would submit my insurance census for the previous day's sessions.

If the session does not happen, it does not mean that the client loses their money. You always have the option of refunding a session and Square makes that very easy. If I become ill and can't perform the session, or the client has a legitimate emergency, I will offer them the option of having a credit for their next session or receiving a refund. Most clients choose to have a credit for their next session, as it can take three to four days for a refund to process back to their card. If a client is having an acute financial crisis, I may, in rare circumstances, decide to provide their session pro bono. There have been situations where I was concerned for my client's safety or they were in danger of relapse, and I felt it was my duty to continue care despite their inability to pay. This system is efficient and effective for myself and the clients, not a heartless business machine that doesn't keep the client's best interests in mind. Over time, you will develop a keen sense of when you need to maintain your boundaries, be flexible, or offer grace.

Chapter Fourteen

Daily Workflow

These daily tasks have remained consistent over the years in my practice. What hasn't remained consistent is my schedule. When I first started my practice and achieved a large client load, I would work ten hours per day, Monday through Friday. For the last several years, I have reduced my schedule to handle projects in my other areas of interest. My schedule is now eight hours per day on Monday, Tuesday, and Thursday. I use Wednesdays as an administrative day to catch up on my reports, court letters, phone calls, and emails. I do my best to take Fridays, Saturdays, and Sundays off. The heavier schedule allowed me to make a serious income and build my assets and savings.

You'll notice that several times throughout the day, I respond to new client emails and voicemails. This is very important, as new clients typically call multiple counselors when seeking help. Whichever counselor calls them back first often gets the new client! If new client calls come in after 7 p.m., I will typically respond to them the following morning. Mondays and Tuesdays tend to be the heaviest days for new client calls. When I first started my practice and calls came in over the weekend, I would quickly respond so as not to lose the client. You should respond to them as quickly as possible when you start out until your caseload reaches the level you desire.

Chapter Fifteen

Client Care Workflow

While the intricacies of my clients' substance abuse are as diverse as the clients themselves, most of the processes remain the same for most cases. Over time, you will find that there is a natural flow to how a client enters and exits your practice. There are many communications and tasks throughout this flow that are identical for every client and situation. I have defined and charted the workflow and created standard templates for each of the communications and processes. This will save you an incredible amount of time in your daily work and improve your communication with clients at all stages of their work with you. The typical client care process, or flow, as I call it, looks like the image on the following page.

For every step in this process, I have created a response voicemail or email, a checklist, a form, a template, or another appropriate tool to ensure you are efficient and effective. We will cover each step in the process in the following chapters. Here are the resources available to you on AddictionPrivatePractice.com:

- Initial client inquiry sample voice and email responses

- Screening call form

- New client welcome email

- New client forms

- New client checklist

- Assessment checklist

- Assessment report template

- Referral sheets

- Recovery plan template

- Progress note template

- Sample client letters and reports

- Termination letter

- Continuing care plan template

Chapter Sixteen

Inquiries, Screening, and Assessment

New Client Inquiries

Your clients will find you via one of your online profiles, your website, or a referral. They will reach out in one of two ways: telephone or email. I've found that most clients prefer to call and speak with me before setting up any appointments. If they don't, I require them to do a brief introduction call so that we can ensure we are a good (and appropriate) fit and screen them. This leads to two outcomes: the client seems appropriate and agrees to move forward, or the client is inappropriate and is referred to other resources. The key elements of the screening call are:

- To determine if the client has a substance abuse problem, and if it is their immediate primary issue

- To understand what the client would like to achieve

- To determine eligibility and appropriateness

- To screen for suicidality, homicidal intention, physical detox symptoms, or psychosis

- To explain the process of how you work with clients (intake, assessment, counseling)

- To explain your scope, costs, and insurance policies

- To answer client questions

- To set up an assessment appointment or provide referrals

Believe it or not, I can accomplish these things in less than thirty minutes with almost every client. You will be able to as well once you practice this method and use it regularly. I never charge clients for this initial introduction call. I prefer to call it an introduction call because, for clients, that sounds much less intimidating than a screening call.

If you receive a high number of inquiries, and the clients are inappropriate or requesting things you don't offer, there is something faulty in your marketing, profiles, or website. If people are calling you because they think you take a type of insurance that you don't or that they can afford your services when they can't, or they are looking for help with a problem outside of your scope of practice, then you must review all of your marketing and communication to figure out where they are getting the wrong information and correct it.

If everything is working as planned, you should receive ten to fifty new client inquiries per month. If you have taken my advanced online profile course on AddictionPrivatePractice.com and implement its strategies, I can almost guarantee you will get that many inquiries.

Most of these new inquiries will not result in a new client; that is normal. If I have ten inquiries in a month, perhaps four will convert to new clients. If I have fifty, it may be twenty new clients. Just because you screen and assess someone does not mean they will become a client. In both steps, I have discovered things that determine the client inappropriate and provide them with referrals. Don't fret about losing clients that aren't appropriate; if you get two, four, or six or more new clients in a month, you are doing excellently! Many of you will do even better than that. Over time, it will build into a very strong practice.

You should respond to new client inquiries as fast as possible. The possibility of a new inquiry converting to a client drops dramatically each hour that passes. If you get two or three days out, they almost never convert. You should also respond to all inquiries. I do my best to respond to every single inquiry, even if I know they are inappropriate. It is the humane thing to do, and it provides many, many referrals to other professionals I work closely with regularly. If you can't help them, give them referrals to people who can. Also, understand that sometimes I was so busy, I just couldn't respond to everyone in a timely fashion or sometimes at all. It cuts down dramatically on new clients when you are that busy, but that usually means you already have enough clients. It is still important to respond to them if you can.

If you have no room for new clients, you can record a separate voicemail stating you are not accepting new clients and that will save your and the prospective clients' precious time. You can also mark your profiles as "*not accepting new clients at this time*" and then change them back when you have openings. Some clients want to be on a waiting list, so I maintain one and call them in order when I have new openings. If your introduction call feels like it is going to run longer than the thirty-minute timeframe, I will focus and redirect the client with a comment like, "*Unfortunately, I only have a limited amount of time for our call today. May I ask you a few more quick questions so that we can cover everything we need to?"*

Screening

Determining whether a client is eligible or appropriate for services is a core function and applies to counselors in private practice. I specifically want to know if there are any obvious signs of suicidality, homicidal intention, psychosis, medical detox symptoms, or coexisting conditions (medical, mental, or physical). The CCAPP ADC Handbook (2017) defines screening as *"The process by which the client is determined appropriate and eligible for admission to a particular program."* While your services in private practice are not a program, screening is still a critical component of what we do every day. The global criteria are:

1. Evaluate the psychological, social, and physiological signs and symptoms of alcohol and other drug abuse.

2. Determine the client's appropriateness for intake or referral.

3. Determine the client's eligibility for intake or referral.

4. Identify any coexisting conditions (medical, psychiatric, physical, etc.) that show the need for additional professional assessment and/or services.

5. Adhere to applicable laws, regulations, and agency policies governing alcohol and other drug abuse services.

Because this is a screening and the assessment seeks to cover in-depth information, I am always looking for obvious signs or data provided by the client. To screen properly, I use questions like:

- Have you seen my website and reviewed the information I provide on my practice?

- Tell me why you reached out to me?

- What happened leading up to your decision to seek help?

- What frequency and quantity have you been drinking or using for the previous two months?

- Are you having any physical withdrawal symptoms right now?

- Have you ever had physical withdrawal symptoms in the past, or do you anticipate any when you stop or cut down?

- Have you been contemplating death recently, or do you feel like hurting someone else?

- Have you had any suicide attempts in the past?

- Are you currently a resident of California?

- Have you ever had, or do you now have, any diagnosis for any medical or mental health condition?

- What medications are you currently taking?

- Do you feel you are seeing or hearing anything that other people don't?

- What is your desired outcome in working with me?

I have found that these questions cover what I need to know in order to properly screen a client. If something serious exists, it doesn't mean they aren't appropriate for counseling. It doesn't mean they absolutely can't work with me. However, it will cause referrals and a request to provide clearance for outpatient substance abuse counseling from another provider. Many clients follow those instructions and come back when they are stable enough to benefit from outpatient counseling. If they aren't appropriate, I will still create a client file in my EMR system, and I document the screening call, referrals, and other information.

Pre-Assessment Activities

If they are appropriate for services, I perform the following pre-assessment activities:

1. Create a client file in the EMR system.

2. Send a setup email from the client portal.

3. Set up electronic screening tools I am using with the client.

4. Review the intake forms and assessment reports before the assessment appointment.

I expect two outcomes before the assessment appointment occurs: that the client completes the new client forms in the EMR system, and completes any electronic assessment tools. Sometimes clients are too high or drunk to complete a screening or an assessment. If so, they usually have a more serious mental health problem or brain damage, or are completely unmotivated to complete these tasks. These situations typically result in a need to refer to a higher level of care, so it is imperative that you investigate the cause.

HerdmanHealth Information

HerdmanHealth offers Behavioral Health Assessment Software that streamlines the assessment process and generates a professional narrative and treatment plan —saving you time and increasing your revenue. Products include Substance Use, Mental Health and Co-occurring evaluations for adults and adolescents and the ASI and ASI-Lite. As part of the Herdman Assessment Forms you can also generate a client Treatment Plan based on the mutually agreed upon problems of the client. The HAF forms include sections on the ASAM-4th Edition to assist in level of care determinations; a section to add collateral information; Problem List (to treat, case manage, or refer); quick access to DSM-5TR diagnostic codes; recommendations; and a treatment plan narrative.

Once a client completes their intake forms, I receive a notification from the EHR system, I proceed with setting up the assessment and email the links to the client. The welcome email covers very important information I want to remind the client of, such as an overview of the process, a friendly reminder on the cancellation policy, the confidentiality law and my mandated reporting requirements, and a reminder that if a client is in crisis, they may call me but that if it is an emergency they should call 911. I also let them know they will receive instruction emails on how to take the online assessments. The assessment email covers instructions on how to take the assessments and the links to do so. If I have not received the required data the night before the appointment, I send them a reminder email and let them know we will have to cancel the appointment if I do not receive it.

When you think about the data from the Herdman assessment, an ASI assessment, and my 90-minute clinical interview—that is a much more comprehensive assessment than almost any client ever receives at a treatment center or outpatient program. Clients feel like I have truly assessed all areas of their substance abuse because I have actually done so, and taken the time to read it and carefully consider their recovery plan. They really appreciate the fact that they didn't simply complete a simple questionnaire and show up and start talking in a session or be forced into a one-size-fits-all program with no concern for their unique story, circumstances, and needs. Technology makes it easy to harness all of this data and use it for the benefit of our clients.

Assessment

The CCAPP ADC Handbook (2017) defines assessment as "*The procedures by which a counselor/program identifies and evaluates an individual's strengths, weaknesses, problems, and needs for the development of a treatment plan.*"

The global criteria for an assessment include:

1. Gather relevant history from the client, including but not limited to alcohol and other drug abuse using appropriate interview techniques.

2. Identify methods and procedures for obtaining corroborative information from significant secondary sources regarding the client's alcohol and other drug abuse and psychosocial history.

3. Identify appropriate assessment tools.

4. Explain to the client the rationale for the use of assessment techniques in order to facilitate understanding.

5. Develop a diagnostic evaluation of the client's substance

abuse and any coexisting conditions based on the results of all assessments to provide an integrated approach to treatment planning based on the client's strengths, weaknesses, and identified problems and needs.

Standard Alcohol and Drug Assessments (Evaluations)

Standard alcohol and drug assessments are non-forensic evaluations. They occur in my practice for three reasons:

- The client would like to receive substance abuse counseling from me.

- The client discontinued counseling over thirty days ago and would like to restart.

- An assessment is needed for help with consultation or treatment placement.

I perform a full alcohol and drug assessment on all new clients. In addition, if a client has seen me for counseling and stopped services for longer than thirty days, I require them to undergo another full assessment. I will not allow a new client to begin counseling without an assessment, as the information provided is essential to a safe and positive outcome. Assessment drives the treatment plan. I inform clients I cannot accept them for counseling services until an assessment is completed. Even though I fully screen clients before they enter my office, there have been cases where I have discovered something in the assessment that results in my referral of the client to another clinician or higher level of care.

In the assessment interview session, I perform the following activities:

- Review state and federal confidentiality laws.

- Explain the reason for and role of the assessment.

- Get releases of information for other providers or programs the client has seen.

- Obtain history in the following areas: medical, physical health, substance abuse, mental health, medications, interpersonal, family, education, career, sociocultural, military, legal, and other relevant data including barriers to treatment, strengths, and coping strategies.

- Review summary data from the HAF and ASI with the client.

- Discuss the criteria for a substance use disorder with the client and which criteria they meet.

- Discuss their goals and vision for their recovery.

- Discuss counseling objectives to achieve these goals.

- Discuss additional services or referrals the client may need to address, such as medical detox, psychiatry, trauma support, or others.

Third-Party Alcohol and Drug Assessments (Evaluations)

Besides standard assessments, I regularly receive clients who need assessments for various court hearings or are mandated to receive one because of a DUI or other crime, by their school, employer, a government agency, licensing or certification board, or a family member. The full assessment gives me the information I need to work with the client to create an assessment report, findings, and recommendations for treatment. Besides the activities above, I require three additional components:

- The client provides all relevant documents related to the current incident or previous ones including police reports, incident reports, drug test results, DMV records, criminal history records, prescription records, medical records, or any other relevant documents.

- The client submits to a laboratory-verified drug and alcohol test (twelve panels or more), the day before, the day of, or the day after their assessment interview. The client submits the results to me as soon as they become available.

- A minimum of five collateral contacts. Collateral contacts are family members, friends, coworkers, supervisors, colleagues, or anyone who has known the client for more than one year. The maximum number of family members is two; the rest must be non-family. If the client has a spouse or significant other, they must be on the list. If there is a prescribing physician involved, no matter how long the client has been using them, I require a release and contact them.

I ask clients to bring the list of collateral contacts to the assessment interview session so that we may review it together and I can screen it for appropriateness before I contact them. You must also have the client sign a release of information for each contact and place it in their file. I can only contact collateral contacts after securing a release, gathering all assessment data, and conducting their interview sessions. When I call the contacts, my primary aim is to corroborate the data the client has reported to me. This is a critical step because, until this point, everything is self-reported by the client. I have had many cases where it appears the client might not have a substance use disorder, and then someone close to them says, "*Well, I really don't want them to know I said this, but I believe they have a problem, or I am very concerned.*"

When you discover new information during the collateral contact process or find out the client has been dishonest or concealed information, it often requires more time than a typical assessment. That is why in my financial agreement and my discussion with the client leading up to the assessment, I inform them that if I discover they have concealed anything, been untruthful, or I have to investigate further because of dishonesty, they are billed at my normal hourly rate for any additional work that needs to be conducted besides my normal assessment fee. If an average assessment takes four hours to complete, and you discover something dishonest that takes an additional four hours to properly investigate, then you need to be compensated for that time.

When interviewing a collateral contact, I fully identify myself to the contact, explain why I am calling and the purpose of the assessment, and inform them I have a release of information to speak with them. I allow them to ask me questions but politely inform them I can't provide any specific information related to the client. I then ask questions such as:

- How long have you known the client?

- What is your relationship with the client?

- Have you ever known this client to have drug or alcohol problems?

- Have you ever been concerned about the client's behavior in any way?

- What have you observed to be this client's typical drinking or use behavior?

- Are you aware of any arrests or emergency room visits this client has had?

These questions may lead to additional questions, but often they do not. If there is a problem with what the client has reported to me, I often notice differences in the details. The length of the relationship or the nature of it is different, incidents are provided that the client never mentioned, additional substances or other types of alcohol, and much more. These things don't mean a client has been dishonest, and sometimes contacts get their information confused. However, if things reported by the contacts felt like something was amiss, I require more collateral contacts. I use a fresh Word document to record my questions and the contact's responses while I am interviewing them. I place these notes in the client's file.

It is necessary to compile all the information collected during the assessment process in a clear and concise manner in the assessment report. For standard assessments, I simply enter the information into my assessment report template and include it in the client's chart. For third-party assessments, I write a formal report on my letterhead and include a copy in the client's chart. Assessments are one of the more time-consuming activities you will conduct in your practice, but also one of the most enjoyable and interesting.

Chapter Seventeen

Recovery Plans & Counseling

Recovery (Treatment) Plans

I refer to treatment plans as recovery plans, as I feel this is a more positive term than "treatment," and clients feel less stigmatized. The CCAPP ADC Handbook (2017) defines treatment planning as the *"process by which the counselor and the client identify and rank problems needing resolution; establish agreed-upon immediate and long-term goals; and decide upon a treatment process and the resources to be utilized."*

The global criteria are:

- Explain the assessment results to the client in an understandable manner.

- Identify and rank problems based on individual client needs in the written treatment plan.

- Formulate agreed-upon immediate and long-term goals using behavioral terms in the written treatment plan.

- Identify the treatment methods and resources to be utilized as appropriate for the individual client.

I discuss the major components of the plan with my clients at the end of the assessment session. This allows me to complete the recovery plan and present it for the client's signature in the first regular counseling session. When discussing the plan components with the client at the end of the assessment session, I use the criteria as my guide to ensure the plan is complete. I never overcomplicate my recovery plans and know that I can always revise or update the plan as needed throughout my work with a client. In my experience, the simpler the plan, the easier it is for a client to see the path forward and achieve the goals.

Counseling

Now that you have screened the client, completed the intake, performed the assessment, and created a recovery plan—it's time to counsel! What do I do during my counseling sessions? I execute the recovery plan, support clients through crises that occur during their counseling, and provide experience, strength, and hope, as they like to say in twelve-step programs.

Counseling, as defined by the CCAPP ADC Handbook (2017), is: *"the utilization of special skills to assist individuals, families, or groups in achieving objectives through exploration of a problem and its ramifications, examination of attitudes and feelings; consideration of alternative solutions; and decision-making."*

The global criteria are:

- Select the counseling theory(ies) that apply(ies).

- Apply technique(s) to assist the client, group, and/or family in exploring problems and ramifications.

- Apply technique(s) to assist the client, group, and/or family in examining the client's behavior, attitudes, and/or feelings if appropriate in the treatment setting.

- Individualize counseling in accordance with cultural, gender, and lifestyle differences.

- Interact with the client in an appropriate therapeutic manner.

- Elicit solutions and decisions from the client.

- Implement the treatment plan.

My counseling sessions typically last forty-five minutes, but I also offer thirty-minute and sixty-minute sessions. There are no predetermined number of sessions or length of the counseling relationship, as they vary from client to client. My clients often have homework or research assignments that prepare them for the next session or strengthen their skills or knowledge in an important area. I cover the global criteria in each core function area throughout the counseling process and properly document sessions in progress notes.

If you haven't used the Wiley Practice Planners before, they are an invaluable resource for any counselor new to private practice. They publish The *Addiction Treatment Planner*, *The Addiction Progress Notes Planner*, and *The Addiction Treatment Homework Planner*. They include over 100 homework assignments, treatment plans, and progress notes for every scenario. You can even print, download, or email the assignments. They have also created planners for many other mental health and behavioral health providers, not just addiction focused providers.

The Herdman Assessment Form (HAF) can also generate for you a treatment (recovery) plan based on the client's Problem List. HerdmanHealth can also assist you in personalizing the treatment plan for your private practice.

Chapter Eighteen

Continuing Care Plans & Termination

Continuing Care Plans

While not one of the twelve core functions, continuing care planning is essential to the success of your clients. In some parts of the country, continuing care planning has actually become a legal requirement in certain treatment scenarios. I believe that having a comprehensive plan for continued care is the most effective approach for counselors and their clients. These plans are also referred to as discharge plans or aftercare plans.

My continuing care plans include:

Identifying areas in which the client needs additional ongoing support.

Identifying ongoing recovery maintenance activities.

Identifying support persons, groups, and activities.

Defining a client's relapse warning signs.

Creating an action plan in the event warning signs become evident.

Creating an action plan in the event a relapse occurs.

I begin continuing care planning several sessions before the intended termination date. I print out the template I have created, bring it to the session, and complete each section with the client. I then encourage the client to digest the contents and reflect on anything we may have missed. We formalize it in the final meeting, and I provide the client with a copy. When conducted correctly, this process creates a feeling of accomplishment and serves as a meaningful conclusion to your work with the client. It creates a very clear path forward and feels like a proper continuation of the journey, not an abrupt termination.

Termination

As shown in the Client Workflow chart, there are typically three ways in which a client discontinues their relationship with their counselor in private practice:

Successful completion.

Repeat no-shows and self-termination.

Referral out to services.

Termination always results in my issuing a termination letter to the client. I typically send this letter by email if the client has communicated with me using email, mail it to their address, or hand it to them in person during their last session.

If a counselor discontinues services to a client who is in need without clearly defining the reason or manner of termination, it can cause premature termination or abandonment. This constitutes malpractice, and the termination letter contains all the components to avoid abandonment. I use three template termination letters for the scenarios listed above that I customize based on the client's needs.

Ideally, proper termination includes:

- Preparing the client for the termination in advance. This provides the client with an opportunity to discuss the termination.

- Referrals may be discussed and prepared for the continuing care plan.

- Avoiding termination communicated by text or voicemail.

- Ensuring the client understands why the relationship is ending, when the termination will occur, and what their next steps are.

- Delivering the termination letter.

- Proper documentation of the termination.

Be sure to include the following in your termination letters:

- Client's name.

- Date counseling began and ended.

- Reasons for termination.

- Recommendations for continuing care or treatment.

- Referral information (three referrals is the standard).

- Write "Confidential" at the top of the letter and do not include any confidential counseling information.

Successful Completion

Every counselor's preferred outcome is when the client has successfully completed the goals of their recovery plan and no further relationship is necessary. It is easy to complete these termination letters, as the continuing care plan already contains the referrals and recommendations. I simply reference the continuing care plan in the termination letter, as there is no need to duplicate the information.

Repeat No-Shows and Self-Termination

As stated in my informed consent for counseling, when a client does not show up for two consecutive sessions, I will attempt to reach out and follow up with the client to determine the reason for the no-shows and whether they would like to continue sessions. I respect the client's wishes and never apply high-pressure sales tactics. If they inform me they are terminating, I will also attempt to follow up. Despite the follow-up attempt, sometimes the client does not respond at all; I then prepare a termination letter and send it to the client. I only make one attempt to reach out to clients, as repeated attempts may be unethical and cause discomfort for the client.

Referrals

This type of termination is often the result of many scenarios but usually requires the same type of termination letter. The scenarios can include, but are not limited to:

- The client does not pay their fees in accordance with the financial agreement (special conditions apply).

- It is determined the client needs a higher level of care or is beyond the counselor's scope of practice.

- The counselor is unwilling to continue care due to threats of violence, a crime committed against the counselor; the counselor feels unsafe, they are closing their practice, retiring, or other appropriate reasons.

- The client fails to participate in counseling.

- The client is not responding to counseling.

When I say that special conditions apply to terminations for non-payment, it is because we have a duty to continue counseling if we did not clearly communicate our financial policies or obtain written agreement to them, if the client is an imminent threat to themselves or others, or if the counselor has failed to discuss the clinical and legal consequences of non-payment prior to termination. As mentioned previously, there are situations in which I will provide pro bono sessions for clients if they are motivated and engaged in their counseling and experience an unexpected financial hardship.

When sending the termination letter, it is important to include the word "Confidential" on the front of the envelope. I have a return address stamp that I use for my practice, which has my address only (no name or other identifying information), and after a line space, "Confidential." If I have not previously discussed the termination letter in the session leading up to termination, I send the letter with delivery confirmation. You can obtain a barcode sticker for delivery confirmation from the post office and add additional postage to receive the notification. You can have a custom return address stamp created by Vista Print.

Chapter Nineteen

Scheduling, Late Cancellations, and Reschedules

S cheduling is something you will do throughout the day, every day. This chapter will discuss the recommended methods for planning and managing appointments, including dealing with last-minute changes or cancellations. Effective scheduling will not only save you time and money but will also decrease downtime and keep your clients happy.

Scheduling Best Practices

I have worked many configurations of days and hours over the years. Some interesting things I have noticed are that clients prefer evenings or weekdays over weekends. With more people working from home with flexible work schedules, it is easier than ever for most clients to do daytime appointments during the workweek. You should maintain a consistent schedule of days and times that you work; otherwise, it will be confusing for clients, and they will miss appointments.

Over the last few years, I have typically worked Monday through Thursday from 10 a.m. to 7 p.m., taking an hour's lunch break. Most clients do not want to come in before 10 a.m., but this time range covers the lunch hour and a few hours after normal working hours, providing opportunities for people with no work flexibility to schedule sessions. It also gives me time in the morning to conduct all the administrative tasks I need to complete, return some calls in the middle of the day, and call back new clients in the evening when it is usually the best time to reach them. Best of all, it keeps me out of rush hour traffic, which can save hours off my day.

When I schedule a new appointment, I first offer times that are before or after my existing appointments or any gaps in between. This keeps my schedule tight and prevents two- or three-hour windows in between sessions. For example, if my schedule for any day were to look like this:

10 a.m. – Empty

11 a.m. – Empty

12 p.m. – Jane Doe

1 p.m. – Empty

2 p.m. – Lunch Hour

3 p.m. – John Doe

4 p.m. – Eric Doe

5 p.m. – Empty

6 p.m. – Kevin Doe

I would initially offer the 1 p.m. and 5 p.m. openings to fill in the gaps. I usually say, "Let's see, I have a 1 p.m. and 5 p.m. open on that day. Will one of those work?" If they don't work for the client, then I would offer the 10 a.m. and 11 a.m. slots. If they can't make a session in any of these openings, we look at another day. I rarely rearrange my appointments with other clients to accommodate one particular client. In the beginning, when your client load is low, I would ask the client what day and time windows work best in the future, then try to find a spot that fits into that and is most convenient for both of you.

If a client can make that appointment regularly, I will put it on the calendar as a recurring appointment for ten weeks. Then I don't have to remember to schedule them for the following week's session, and when I'm looking at later dates on my calendar, I don't accidentally schedule someone in their spot. In addition, I have my EMR system (SimplePractice) configured to send a reminder email two days before the session and a text message one day before the session. Reminders significantly cut down on missed appointments and make it fair and easy to enforce your cancellation policy. My clients can respond to the automated reminders if they need to cancel, and it automatically changes their appointment status in my calendar.

Late Cancellations and Reschedules

Strict enforcement of your cancellation and reschedule policy will help you and your clients. It helps your clients to be accountable and engaged in their counseling. Keeping appointments and following the rules are important habits most people with substance abuse problems struggle with. Modeling appropriate boundaries with these behaviors prevents you from enabling your client. If a client is habitually late or misses appointments frequently, there is often something else going on that needs to be explored. This can be a symptom of ADHD or other problems, and this behavior can actually lead to relapses. Proper boundary setting will also save you thousands of dollars per year and many wasted hours.

Since you are charging the clients scheduled that day in the morning, anyone who has not canceled or rescheduled by that time is clearly in violation of the policy. I give clients one free pass on no-shows, late canceling, or the late rescheduling of an appointment. It's okay if you don't, and I don't mention this in my cancellation policy as I don't want clients to expect it. I have found that the first time this happens, extending some grace and reinforcing the policy can strengthen the counseling relationship, not weaken it. I usually say something like, "It's unfortunate you weren't able to make your appointment. As you know from our financial agreement, I do charge clients for the session if they miss it or late cancel. However, I'm willing to give you one free pass on this if you can commit to keeping these to a minimum and you understand that for any future no-shows, I must charge you." Clients appreciate this gesture and usually take the policy seriously in the future.

In situations where there is a verifiable emergency, such as an ER visit for their child, a car accident, or a death in the family, I will waive the cancellation policy fee if they can provide some proof of the incident. These are situations in which a client has no control and did not create the incident, but such situations are also very rare. With these policies in place, overall, I don't have many clients miss appointments, and my week usually works out as planned, including my expected income. If you have a hard time enforcing your cancellation policy, it may be a good idea to explore potential codependency issues and work on them.

Chapter Twenty

Referrals

I provide referrals to clients daily: are not appropriate for my services, who need additional resources, or if they are terminated. If you have to look up referrals, copy their contact information, write them down, or compose a custom email with this information—it is very time consuming. Because it is so time consuming, you may fail to provide as many referrals or as thorough a list of options as you should.

I have created a system I call *"Referral Sheets"* that has served my clients and myself well over the years. When I need to make a referral, I give my clients a referral sheet for the resources they need. I keep them in hard copy in my office and in electronic format so I can quickly email them. While these referral sheets take some time and effort to create, they will save you so much time and money that it is essential to create them. Here are the referral sheets I maintain with contact information for local:

- Psychiatrists

- Psychologists

- MFTs

- LPCCs

- Addiction Physicians

- Medical Detox Facilities

- Treatment Programs (Residential, IOP)

- Trauma Specialists

- ADHD Specialists

- Drug Testing Locations

- Free and Low-Cost Treatment Services

- 12-Step Meetings (separate sheets for men, women, young adults)

- LGBTQ Meetings and Resources

- Non-12-Step Support Groups (Smart Recovery, Recovery Dharma, Women for Sobriety, and more)

- Religious Support Groups

- Gambling Disorders (CalGETS, NCPG, Clinicians, Programs)

- Family Resources (MFTs, Support Groups, Al-Anon, CODA, ACOA)

- Recovery-Related Books

- Sober Living Environments and Emergency Shelters

- Attorneys (Criminal, Family Law)

- Planned Parenthood and STD Testing

This may seem like a lengthy list, but I use all of them regularly. If I did not have them, I would have to compile them every time I needed them. I do my best to have four or five resources in each area. Unfortunately, there may not be that many, but if there are only one or two, that is better than zero, so it is important to list them. There is a sample referral sheet on the website, and the data I typically include are the name, address, phone, website, and email of the resource. I also do my best to list whether they take insurance and what their rates are. I get that information by calling them and letting them know I'd like to include them as a referral resource and need some basic information to give my clients. This opens the door to a professional relationship with these resources, and if possible, I will request more information or set up a tour. It also helps you get noticed by them, and they might start recommending you to others.

If a client isn't appropriate for my services, I say, "*Let me send you some referrals in an email really quick so you can find the help you need.*" I attach the referral sheets and send them. Done in 30 seconds! If a client repeatedly does not show or self-terminates, I send them a termination letter or email and include the referral sheets with it. When I discuss the need for additional resources with clients, I never have to say, "*Let me look into some referrals and get back to you*" or "*Go home and Google,*" I just hand it right to them, and we can both get on with our day! Be sure to document in a client's file whenever you provide them with referrals of any type. On the progress note template provided on the website, I have included a section where you can list any referral sheets given during a session.

IMPORTANT UPDATE: I now have a tool available on AddictionPrivatePractice.com that instantly creates referral sheets for you in your area on every topic listed above. What would normally take hours or days to create now only takes minutes.

Chapter
Twenty-One

Crisis Calls & High-Risk Clients

I n twelve years as an addiction counselor, I've had to make several calls to 911 and one report to child protective services. They are not as frequent as you might expect, but they happen. Knowing how to handle these clients and situations is critical to protecting your clients, yourself, and ensuring the best possible outcome.

What is a High-Risk Client?

I consider a high-risk client to be any client who has a major mental health or medical issue beyond my scope of practice, besides a substance abuse problem. Some examples of co-occurring issues that may be high-risk are:

- Schizophrenia

- Bipolar disorder

- Borderline personality disorder

- Suicidal ideation

- Pre-detox and physically dependent

- Major depressive disorder

- Late-stage liver problems

- Life-threatening medical issues

- Unresolved or triggered PTSD or sexual trauma

There are more conditions, but these are the most common I encounter in private practice. In scenarios where a client presents with one of these conditions, or I suspect they may have one, I require one of two things: (1) the client is under the care of a medical or mental health professional and provides me with a written release of information; or (2) the client finds a medical or mental health professional to diagnose or treat their condition and provides me with a written release of information. I may require a doctor's note clearing them for outpatient counseling if they have a serious or potentially life-threatening medical condition.

As part of the new client paperwork, I have already had them sign a release of information for an emergency contact. I remind them of this release and ask if this is still the best person to reach out to if I can't contact them and am concerned about their safety. If they have a new or better contact, I will ask them to update the release with the new information.

I then reach out to the medical or mental health professional to let them know I am working with their patient and coordinate care. I inform the client that they must secure this care before I can work with them, and/or that they must continue this care for the duration of our counseling. To be successful in recovery, a client must address all the conditions listed above. Their substance abuse must usually stop before they can recover from any of these conditions. This becomes a treatment team scenario where I collaborate with their other medical or mental health professionals to ensure a positive outcome. I follow the medical or mental health professional's instructions and collaborate; I never advise my clients to do anything against medical advice.

One of the biggest indicators of suicidality or major depressive disorder that I have noticed over the years in my practice is when a client breaks down emotionally in their initial inquiry message, screening call, or assessment. They try to tell you information and burst into tears, unable to get it all out. Many times, such clients have later admitted that they were suicidal after receiving proper treatment for their major depressive episode. Proper referrals in these types of scenarios will ensure the best possible outcome for your client. I often request that the client check in with me each day until they have secured help, begun treatment, and stabilized. You never want to hope they pull out of it in these scenarios. Compassionately require they get the help they need, and support them through the process. If they are suicidal, you must take immediate action.

Crisis Calls

I receive about one serious after-hours crisis call every six months. These often involve:

- A major relapse

- A major shift in mental status such as suicidality, major depression, or panic attacks

- The death of a loved one

- An imminent threat of relapse because of a car accident, layoff, criminal charges, or other major incidents

- Significant medical diagnosis

- Psychotic break

- Client under the influence

- Possible overdose

- Served with divorce papers or another type of lawsuit

Again, these are just a few examples of the crisis calls I receive. I created a crisis response worksheet for these scenarios, which is available to you on the AddictionPrivatePractice.com website. I use this worksheet as I am working through the crisis. This helps to ensure I don't miss any critical steps or information, and I also then have complete documentation for the client's file. The components of handling crisis calls effectively include safety, communication, referrals, follow-up, and documentation.

Safety

Your priority in a crisis is to determine if they need an emergency services response. Knowing where your client is physically located is important if your client will disclose that information. If a client calls and I don't answer, and they leave a voicemail like *"I just can't go on anymore and I'm going to kill myself*" then hang up—I call 911. I follow the instructions of the emergency services dispatcher regarding whether I should attempt to contact the client. I provide 911 with whatever information they need to locate them. With present technology, if a client has a mobile phone with them and it is on, they can often locate them quickly.

If I answer the call and they tell me the same thing in real-time, I will attempt to determine their location, support them, and summon emergency services if needed. I say things like *"I'm really sorry to hear you are hurting and I'm here to help. Are you at home right now?"* or *"For safety reasons, I need to know where you are."* I also say things like, *"I know you are feeling terrible, but this is temporary, and we can work through this. I'm here to support you."* Familiarize yourself with the best ways to respond to a suicidal client. I needed a refresher in private practice, and there are many great articles online from professionals who specialize in this. These situations are intense, and our brains may not recall information that we need to respond appropriately. That's why I wrote them on my crisis response worksheet.

Other examples of major safety concerns beyond suicidality are psychosis, overdose, detox symptoms, or operating a motor vehicle under the influence.

Communication

If someone leaves me a voicemail and it sounds serious, I do not delay in calling them back. If I have practice coverage in place while I am on vacation, then I let my covering counselor respond. Minutes or hours can sometimes be the difference between life and death. I clearly state in my voicemail message, client forms, and on my website that I do not handle emergency calls—but they will happen, anyway. To ignore them is negligence and can lead to serious liability issues.

It is inevitable, however, that these calls may go unanswered for some period. Especially if I receive the call after I fall asleep and don't receive my messages until the morning. Whenever there has been a significant amount of time between the message and my response, I always call the client back as soon as possible. If I can't reach the client and I believe their life is in danger, I call 911. If it seems serious but not imminently life-threatening, I will call their emergency contact and attempt to locate them and connect.

Following up on a crisis call can be extremely inconvenient, but if you cannot do so in a timely manner, to a client, it feels like their counselor does not care. It's not only dangerous but can add fuel to the fire. If you cannot reach your client or connect with their emergency contact, you can request that the police do a *"welfare check"* to ensure your client is safe. Ask them to have the officer follow up with you on the disposition of the response. If you don't hear from the police officer in a reasonable amount of time, call the police department back and ask about the outcome of the call.

Welfare checks work wonders in a variety of situations. If your client is so high or drunk that they can't properly communicate, or you fear an overdose—request a welfare check. If they are psychotic, delusional, or depressed to the point of serious concern, a welfare check is appropriate. There are many less serious scenarios where I did not have to request a welfare check because the client agreed to allow me to speak to their emergency contact. I contacted that person, and they could monitor the client until help arrived or drive them to get the appropriate services. There are also scenarios where I've contacted an emergency contact and they did not seem capable of managing the situation or were high or drunk themselves. In those situations,

I request a welfare check. To provide you with a reference point on how often I must request welfare checks, last year I had to request no welfare checks and most years are the same.

Emergency Room Referrals

When it comes to emergency rooms, if I tell someone they need to go to the emergency room, particularly if they are in acute detox, I don't just tell them to go and then hope it all works out. Have you ever sent a client in acute detox to an emergency room (ER)? It can be a disturbing experience. Often, when a client goes to the ER, medical professionals label them as an alcoholic or addict, and they frequently receive minimal treatment, lack access to resources, and sometimes face shame. I was deeply concerned and discouraged the first few times this happened. It can be extremely demoralizing for a client when they are trying to do the right thing. It's sad, but it happens thousands of times every day across the country.

ERs constantly deal with medication-seeking addicts, overdoses, and alcohol poisoning. It creates compassion fatigue. When they understand someone is trying to recover and is working with a professional, it can make all the difference. I have developed a solution that virtually works every time a client is headed to the ER. I inquire with the client if they would like me to call the ER while they are en route, providing them with a heads-up regarding their situation and our objectives. By letting them know, I am often successful in enlisting the ER's support. The clients usually agree, I have them sign a release (often electronically), and I call the ER immediately. Here is how that conversation usually starts:

"Hello, I'm Michael O'Brien. I'm an Addiction Counselor and I have a client who is on their way to the emergency room. His name is John

Doe, and he is a 50-year-old Asian male. His wife is driving him. The reason I referred him is that he is having acute detox symptoms and I'm concerned for his safety. He reported heavy sweating, tremors, and he hasn't been able to eat for over 24 hours. He seems very dehydrated. I just wanted to give you guys a heads-up and also let you know John is seeking help and working with a professional. He underestimated how serious his withdrawal symptoms would be, but he is motivated to work a program of recovery. Is there any other information you need from me?"

They will usually ask questions about how long he has been drinking, how much, when did he stop, and I provide them with any information they need. It's amazing how much this simple phone call can transform an ER visit for a client. Clients often say, *"Wow! They treated me like a VIP when I walked in and they were really caring and fixed me right up!"* Spending less than five minutes to make this call can mean the difference between success and failure for your client. I have never had a hospital be anything but professional and appreciative when I've made these calls.

Is this being codependent? I don't believe it is. It's coordinating care, advocating for your client, and doing your best to ensure a positive outcome. The entire system works better when we all communicate.

Follow-Up

We can never just assume everything turned out alright when a crisis call occurs. Most of my crisis calls do not require the police, EMT, or emergency contacts. I'm thankful when they don't. But in almost all crisis scenarios, I always follow up with a client. If a client has relapsed and calls late at night, I will do my best to make sure they are safe and can restart their recovery the next day. I always ask if it is OK for me to reach out to them the next day and make sure they are doing better. Sometimes I will set up a follow-up session within a few days if they can make it into the office. If they go to the hospital or a detox facility, I ask them if it is alright to call them there and check on them.

The purpose of following up is not to be annoying or intrusive, it's about safety and compassion. If possible, I always ask for permission. Then I put a reminder on my calendar to do a follow-up, and avoid possibly forgetting and disappointing my client. These calls are often uplifting for clients and boost their spirits. However, sometimes they help the client avoid disaster. On many follow-up calls, I have heard things like *"I love this place, but I just found out my insurance won't cover it, I don't know what to do"* or *"I'm so stressed out because I am missing work and don't know how to handle it."* There are many situations where you can help your client move through what seems to be a major obstacle and guide them in resolving a problem or continuing care somewhere else.

Documentation

There is one last step that is just as important as the others—documentation. It is critical that you properly document your response to crisis calls. Think of it as a progress note with all the information on what happened and what the outcome was. You should document:

- The date, time, and reason for the crisis

- All of your actions including, initial response, referrals, follow-up calls, and emergency contacts

- The client's response to your actions

- The outcome and follow-up plans

If you use the crisis response form that I have created, you will document these things and not forget anything important. This documentation isn't only required; it is critical in the event your actions ever come into question. Many counselors want to overthink this because of the severity of the situation, but a simple, clear, concise report is sufficient. If I am adding information to the form as I go along, I can usually finish it in just a few brief minutes. You can forward voicemails, text messages, or emails to your secure email and then include them in the client's chart.

Chapter Twenty-Two

Returning Clients

As addiction is a chronic and progressive illness, some clients may relapse after long periods of success. I've had clients who have been clean for six months, two years, and even five years relapse and seek my services again. There is a lot of shame and guilt surrounding relapses after long periods of sobriety, so it's an honor that clients trust me enough and valued their previous experience enough to return. Once you have seen hundreds of clients, some will occasionally come back.

When treated professionally and with compassion, many of these clients can recover quickly and rarely need as many counseling sessions as before. However, if the client has not seen me in over thirty days, I require another full assessment. This is because a lot can change in thirty days, six months, or even years. Clients may develop addictions to different substances, encounter major mental health or medical problems, or face new triggers and stressors. It is important to fully understand what has changed and what led to the relapse. We have a duty to perform another thorough evaluation.

Whenever a client completes services with me, or even if they leave unexpectedly, I always encourage them to return if needed. I let them know while relapse can happen to the strongest in recovery; it doesn't have to be the end of their progress. The genuine tragedy is when people continue using and spiral downward over weeks or months. I tell them I won't judge them and that we'll focus on getting them back on their feet quickly, hopefully preventing any further relapses. I also encourage them to call me even if they don't want to see me again but need a referral to another clinician, medical detox, residential, or intensive outpatient treatment (IOP).

Chapter
Twenty-Three

Impaired Clients

In our line of work, it's inevitable—clients will show up at our offices impaired by drugs or alcohol. As outlined in the informed consent and my new client welcome email, I cover what will happen if a client shows up impaired. Clients are in a dangerous state when they show up under the influence; they have totally lost control of their use. They are experiencing a lot of pain, shame, and guilt, and they can't stop using long enough to come in for a session. This significant indicator of severity should be taken seriously.

Clients usually require medical detox or residential treatment when this occurs, as it is a powerful indicator that they need a higher level of care. There are several ways in which this might happen. A client may be dishonest about their level of use in your initial screening call and show up to the assessment impaired. A client can be strong in their recovery for months, suddenly relapse, conceal it between appointments, and show up impaired. Driving to and from sessions, or entering and leaving the office might be life-threatening. It can be highly disturbing to other clients they may come into contact with, and they can be seriously emotionally unstable. It's not a question of whether this will happen in your practice, but when.

My response to these scenarios is compassionate, with the goal of getting the client safely back home or to the emergency room. It's one or the other; there usually are no other options. I feel it is inappropriate during these scenarios to try to convince a client to enter a higher level of care immediately. The risk of developing or escalating negative emotions is too high. I never shame them, try to teach them a lesson, or "*raise their bottom*." I feel compassion for them, and that is what they need in these moments. It is also the best way to ensure they do not further decline in their emotional state, use more, or hurt themselves or someone else.

Protocol for Managing Impaired Clients

Acknowledgment and Compassionate Conversation: I let the client know compassionately that I've noticed they're not themselves during the session and mention their impairment. I make it comfortable and safe for them to be honest with me about their state of impairment.

Policy Discussion and Medical Assistance: I then discuss my policy on being impaired in session. I let them know that I ethically can't continue a session if they are impaired and ask if they need medical help. If they request medical assistance, or if they are so impaired that they cannot respond or answer questions, I call 911 immediately. If they refuse medical assistance, I still advise them to get checked out and go to the emergency room after they leave.

Transportation Arrangements: If they will be leaving in anything other than an ambulance, I inform them that if they drove to their session, they won't be able to drive home on their own. I tell them that if they attempt to drive home on their own; I am required to report that to the authorities. I ask if there is a friend or family member they trust we could call together on speakerphone to arrange for them to be picked up immediately. Remember that if you need to speak to anyone other than the police or emergency responders, you must remember confidentiality and obtain releases of information. It is important to record the name and contact information of the person picking up the client.

Rideshare or Taxi Service: You always have the options of a rideshare or taxi service. This isn't my preferred method, as the client is then in the hands of someone they don't know. Unfortunately, in very rare circumstances, it is the only option. I've always gone with the client to the vehicle, write down the license plate, and ensured they departed safely.

Documentation: I then document all the facts of the incident in a progress note in their chart. It's important to include the facts about what the client reported using or drinking, whether they declined or accepted medical assistance, if they were instructed to get medical attention after they left, what type of transportation they had, the contact information of the driver or the license plate, and if they left the premises safely in a progress note in their chart. Detailed documentation and charting are essential to protecting yourself from liability.

Follow-Up: I follow up with clients to make sure they are safe, not spiraling further down after the incident, and to discuss the next steps. Sometimes I follow up within an hour or a day, depending on the severity of the situation. Occasionally, I will follow up within a few hours of the incident to make sure the client is safe, then decide when to follow up again to discuss the next steps. Most often, I am working with the client to transition them to a higher level of care or detox, but that isn't the predetermined outcome. This is when your experience in helping clients determine what is best for them really makes a difference. Handled professionally, these situations can really help the client break through denial and take the steps to overcome their addiction.

Chapter Twenty-Four

Mandated Clients

O ver the years, many of my clients have been mandated to complete a substance evaluation, counseling, drug testing, or all three. While the term is commonly used for clients who are ordered to treatment by a criminal court, I consider a mandated client to be any client who requires my services for legal or employment reasons. There are many scenarios outside of the legal system that require clients to use my services, such as professional board violations (for nurses, therapists, counselors, dentists, and more), child custody disputes, a positive random drug test at work, and many more. There are two priorities: the duty to protect public safety, and providing the best possible care for your client.

Protecting public safety is a serious responsibility. How would you feel if you evaluated someone and then they hurt someone else because they didn't get proper treatment or sentencing? You'd feel terrible! These mandated scenarios introduce a sensitive dynamic to the counseling relationship: your duty to protect the public and your duty to help your client. It can create difficult conversations when your client does not agree with your recommendations. It requires that you put aside any need for approval and do what is right despite the pressure from the client or the agency requesting the services. While we would like to think our need for approval never interferes with our work, caring for mandated clients will challenge this area of your psyche. This is normal; consult with your clinical supervisor when these scenarios arise and keep learning and growing.

These are just a few scenarios I've encountered with mandated clients:

- A client had a DUI out-of-state and requires an evaluation to regain their license.

- A client committed a crime while under the influence, and their attorney feels an evaluation will benefit their defense.

- A client is convicted of a crime and is required by a court to complete an evaluation, counseling, or drug testing.

- A client has applied for a professional license such as nursing, commercial airline pilot, or truck driver, and a previous conviction for a crime committed under the influence comes up in a background check; the agency requests an evaluation to rule out active addiction.

- A family court judge orders a parent to receive substance abuse counseling and be monitored daily for alcohol abuse.

- A college student is involved in a substance-related incident or is failing classes and cites substance abuse as a problem;

the college orders an evaluation and requires the student to follow the recommendations.

I have had mandated cases that have made national news because of the crimes of my clients. I follow one simple rule for all of my evaluations: If the client has a substance abuse problem, that is what my report will reflect; if they don't, then it will reflect that they do not. I look at the evidence, and I base my findings and recommendations on that evidence and nothing else.

Many clients have sought my services after being ordered to attend a specific number of sessions or weeks of counseling. These requirements have been as high as fifty sessions or one year of weekly counseling, but most often are under twenty sessions. These clients must participate in substance abuse counseling regardless of my initial assessment or whether I believe they need counseling. It's difficult to have fifty sessions with someone who doesn't actually have a substance abuse problem, but it is rare that they don't. If they don't have a substance use disorder, I focus on education on topics like the effects of substances on the brain, the physical body, how they impair us, and other relevant topics to ensure these sessions are beneficial and serve the spirit of the requirement. In mandated scenarios, clients must make up missed sessions and complete the required amount, whether they want to or not.

To protect public safety in mandated cases, I do several things differently from regular cases:

Identity Verification: A copy of a government-issued photo ID in addition to my standard client paperwork to ensure their identity.

Release of Information: Require the client to sign a release of information for the agency that ordered treatment.

Legal Documents: A copy of all legal documents related to the case.

Collateral Contacts: For assessments, I require a minimum of five, but preferably ten or more, collateral contacts; the majority should be non-family.

Drug and Alcohol Testing: Conduct a lab-verified drug and alcohol test on the day the assessment is conducted.

12-Step Group Attendance: If required to attend 12-step groups, a signed release to speak with their sponsor and a meeting signature card.

Transparency: Inform the client that I have a responsibility to be honest and protect public safety in our first appointment.

Review Requirements: Review the actual order and requirements for the assessment or counseling to ensure I meet the requirements and the services I provide satisfy the order.

Additional Documentation: In some cases, require clients to provide a criminal conviction report, medical records, DMV driving records, or prescription records.

I don't predict or promise any outcomes as they relate to assessments. I inform clients I review all the data collected and typically make recommendations based on accepted standards. Many clients don't understand the exact requirements, so it is important to review the mandated service requirements before commencing any services or assessments to be sure you are the right one for the case. If in doubt, verify with the court or agency any vague or nonspecific requirements. For example, if a client is ordered to attend twenty-five counseling sessions, can they do two or three per week, or just one per week? I don't allow clients to stack their sessions or have one every day until the requirement is met. I allow the client to have as many sessions per week as we agree are necessary and reasonable. Usually, that is one session per week, with more critical clients at two per week, and very severe clients at three sessions per week until they stabilize.

If they are required to attend AA meetings, do they have to provide proof with a signature card? I have seen many cases where a client has gone off and done a bunch of things only to find out they didn't do something correctly, have the wrong type of professional, or fail to properly document what they did. Be very clear about the details of the requirements. In an assessment, I do not recommend that a client must see me for services. I provide them with three referrals for the services they need. If a client requests I work with them and I feel it will be beneficial to them, I will work with them. It is unethical to recommend a client to treatment where a conflict of interest exists. In some scenarios, like SAP evaluations, it is forbidden by law except under very unique circumstances to refer someone to your own services.

> You will find sample reports and letters for mandated clients on the AddictionPrivatePractice.com website.

Chapter Twenty-Five

Time-Off &
Slowdowns

Time Off and Slowdowns

Holidays and vacation time are critical to self-care, avoiding burnout, and preventing compassion fatigue. Clients understand you need time away and will expect you to take time off for vacations, holidays, or family emergencies. In this chapter, we'll discuss how to handle illness, emergency time off, vacations, holidays, and the natural slowdowns that occur throughout the year.

Illness and Family Emergencies

Illness and family emergencies happen; they're a fact of life. When I come down with the flu or a serious cold, I immediately notify my clients that day that I cannot attend our session because of illness. If I get sick in the evening and I'm fairly sure I won't be able to make my sessions the next day, I notify them that night. I typically do this with a text message, as an email may not be seen in time, and a phone call may result in a longer conversation. If you haven't billed your clients for the day or the next day, you don't have to worry about credits or refunds.

Sometimes, I have billed clients in the morning and then come down with a serious fever several hours later. My schedule is often so busy that it is almost impossible to reschedule that day's clients within the same week. The optimal outcome is usually to see the client at the same time next week. If you have already charged them, give them credit and don't charge for the next session. My texts to the affected clients usually look something like this:

"Hi [Client's Name], regrettably, I have come down with a fever and cannot make our session this week. I am unsure how many days I may be out, so resuming at our normal time next week is preferable. However, if you really need to see me, I can let you know if I have any other session times open this week when the illness passes. I had billed all of my clients this morning before the symptoms became obvious, so there will be no charge for your next session. If you prefer, I am also happy to void the charge, but it may take three or four days to post to your card. Let me know how you'd like to handle the schedule and if you'd like a refund today. Thanks! Michael O'Brien."

The response to this text is usually something like, *"I'm sorry you're sick! Hope you feel better soon. Yes, next week is fine, and the credit sounds like the easiest option. See you next week!"* Once all the clients have responded, I can relax and get as much rest as possible. If someone doesn't respond within an hour or two, I will call them and leave a voicemail to ensure I have done my best to notify them. This process works well for almost any scenario in which you need to take unexpected time off.

Vacations or Extended Time Off

I take weeklong vacations throughout the year and have had medical issues requiring surgery, which incapacitated me for weeks. In the weeks before my leave, I remind all clients at the end of our session that I will be gone and what to do in an emergency while I'm away. As after-hour emergencies are rare in private practice, if I am on vacation but in a location where I am totally connected to cellular and internet service, I do not arrange for coverage of my clients with another counselor.

However, I often go *"off the grid"* on my vacations. For off-the-grid vacations, or if it is surgery or another medical reason, I arrange for a counselor with whom I have a transfer plan in place to be available to my clients. I give my clients her contact information the week before I'm away. This counselor will then charge the same fees I do for any work she must undertake with my clients, and those fees are hers to keep.

Holidays and Slowdown Periods

There is a pattern with holidays. In the weeks leading up to a major holiday like Christmas, Thanksgiving, or New Year's, calls from prospective new clients may decrease dramatically, if not to zero. Then, often immediately after the holiday, usually the following day, I receive many new client calls. I believe this is because most people who have a substance abuse problem don't want to quit right before a major holiday. There is much more family tension, alcohol use, and loneliness, all of which spike around the holidays. There are also heightened DUI enforcement and more domestic violence arrests, which result in more assessments or mandated counseling clients.

When I first started my practice, I thought I would be very busy during the holidays because clients would relapse more often. While relapses occur more frequently during the holidays, I've found that if I work with clients on handling potential issues in the weeks leading up to the holidays, it dramatically cuts down on relapses. Even with a client load of thirty or forty clients, I've had Christmases come and go with no client relapses. I dedicate a lot of session time to planning for and managing these holidays with clients before they sneak up on them.

Because of this pattern, I can take off the week when a major holiday occurs, such as the entire week of Christmas, or from Christmas to New Year's, or the entire week of Thanksgiving. If you try to work during these weeks, you will find almost no new client calls, and many clients cancel their sessions the day before because they are too busy with holiday preparations or travel. Use this time to recharge and be with your family and friends. Just prepare your clients for the holidays in advance, and things are typically calm.

The slowest times of the year, which seem consistent every year, are the two weeks before the 4th of July, most of August because of summer vacations, and the two weeks right before Thanksgiving and Christmas. This doesn't mean you will be slow during those times; if your caseload is heavy, those clients will continue to see you leading up to the holiday week. However, new client calls may subside significantly.

January 2nd is often the busiest for new client calls, as people often create New Year's resolutions or like to time their sobriety at the beginning of the year. I never schedule time off during January, as it is one of the busiest months of the year. I take off any federal holidays and popular non-federal holidays like Halloween. Clients tend not to want to have sessions on these days. When I first started out, I would schedule sessions on these days, only to have most of the clients cancel a few days before when they realized they didn't want to come in on Halloween night, Cinco De Mayo, or Valentine's Day. You can see clients on these days, but I would double-check with them the week before to make sure they aren't over-committing themselves.

Biggest Relapse Holidays

Year after year, the number one relapse holiday for my clients has always been the 4th of July, followed by New Year's Eve, Valentine's Day, Cinco De Mayo, and St. Patrick's Day, in that order. This surprised me at first, but I realized clients tend to have more incentive to stay sober on holidays when they spend more time with family. The major relapse holidays are ones where clients spend more time with friends and are more celebratory than religious holidays.

Chapter Twenty-Six

Security

Prioritizing Security in Your Practice

I cannot emphasize enough the importance of being aware of your security at all times, especially when working in private practice. While my clients are amazing people with good intentions when they're clean and sober, they can have severely impaired judgment when they're not. They can become psychotic and impaired, and act out of character. Throughout my career, I have faced several security-related issues that have prompted me to take security seriously and become overly cautious.

Former clients have stalked me on more than one occasion. I worked at a program where a client brutally murdered a mentor and fellow counselor I worked with at a program. I have received threatening phone calls from angry spouses when they don't get what they want in family court. Clients who have relapsed have approached late at night in parking lots and asked for money. These are serious situations in which my safety was at risk. They are rare and not meant to scare you, but to show that we can do our jobs diligently, with the utmost professionalism, and still face instances where we are unjustly the targets of another person's pathology.

We can never be sure when something bad will happen. I consciously think through my security in various areas of my life to be as prepared as possible if something goes wrong. I ask myself questions like: If a client were to attack me in my office, how would I escape or summon help? What if a client relapsed and confronted me in the parking lot when I was leaving at night? What would I do if someone broke into my home while I was there? You may never fully prevent something like that from happening, but if you can summon help, escape, or barricade yourself until help arrives, you improve your odds of survival. Think through these scenarios and have a plan in mind.

It should go without saying that clients should never know your home address. I guard this information with the utmost secrecy. What extra precautions can you take to ensure your safety?

Safety Precautions

Install a Home Security System: Install a security system in your home and place panic buttons in areas where you can easily access them and remain as safe as possible while waiting for help to arrive. I recommend the Ring security system because it is affordable, easy to set up, and has a low monthly monitoring cost. I have a collapsible fire ladder under the bathroom sink in the master bedroom of my two-story home. In the event of a fire or intruder, I can lock myself in the bathroom, press the panic button, and easily escape through the window if necessary. Without these precautions, the outcome of such emergencies could be much worse.

Office Security System: If you have your own office, consider installing a Ring security system there as well. The key fob comes with a panic button that often works from the parking lot. You can also place a panic button under your desk. If you share an office, discuss a security system with the other clinicians. This also adds a layer of security if you store any client files in your office.

Trust Your Instincts: Always trust your instincts. If you feel uncomfortable working with a client in the evening hours or when you are at the office alone, switch their appointment to a time when someone else is in the office or during the day. You can also ask a colleague, friend, or family member to expect a call or text from you at a certain time if you anticipate a difficult situation. If they don't hear from you at the expected time, they can try to contact you and call the police if they cannot reach you. Alternatively, you can refer out a client who you feel may pose a risk to your personal safety.

Install a Security Camera: Consider installing a security camera in your office. Although I initially opposed security cameras in treatment environments due to privacy concerns, I now recognize that they serve as an excellent deterrent for potential criminal activity or false accusations. With advancements in technology, there are now inexpensive cameras that can record weeks of video, and you can disable the audio to ensure further confidentiality.

Add a clause to your informed consent to inform clients about the camera's existence and it not recording audio to protect their confidentiality. Of the hundreds of clients I have seen in my private office with a security camera installed, I've never received a complaint or had a client stop services due to the camera. I place it near the ceiling on the wall behind where my clients sit, and it records the back of their head and the front of me during sessions. Since the camera is behind them, they aren't staring at it throughout the session, and after the first visit, it is almost invisible to them. I check the camera every thirty days to ensure it is functioning properly.

Report Crimes or Threats: Report any criminal activity or threats against you to the police immediately. While it may be unpleasant, documenting the activity can provide a serious deterrent to the perpetrator if the police begin investigating. It can also prevent the same or worse scenarios from happening to someone else or another counselor.

Enhance Digital Security: Use all additional security options available to you. Most online accounts now offer two-factor authentication; turn it on for all practice-related accounts. Ensure you have up-to-date virus and intrusion software on your computer. Use VPN software to encrypt everything you do online. If you don't have a password set up to access your phone, set one up right away. These additional measures make it much more difficult for someone to hack into your life or access client information.

Being vigilant about your security is crucial in our line of work. Implementing these precautions can significantly enhance your safety and ensure you are prepared for any potential threats.

Chapter Twenty-Seven

Drug Testing & Monitoring

Drug Testing & Monitoring

As I mentioned earlier, I do not require clients to undergo drug testing unless it is mandated by a third party. Clients may also request drug testing, or we might add it to their recovery plan if we feel it will be beneficial. There are many scenarios where a third party may require the client to be drug tested randomly, on a schedule, or continuously monitored for a period of time. If these cases involve the criminal justice system, child custody, or affect their freedom, I require them to use a laboratory or the Soberlink system for testing.

Point of Care (POC) Drug Tests

I keep one or two cases of POC drug tests on hand to test clients in the office. Families or clients often purchase tests to take home and administer themselves. While urine drug tests used to be the only option for POC drug tests, science has advanced greatly, and oral fluid (saliva-based) drug tests are now just as reliable and cover as many substances as urine tests. Oral fluid tests allow counselors or loved ones to administer the test in front of them, significantly reducing the ability to alter the test results. They are also less embarrassing for the client. I use oral fluid tests manufactured to forensic standards to ensure their accuracy. If a client tests positive with either a urine or saliva test and there could be legal consequences, I have the positive result verified by a laboratory.

When administering POC drug tests, standard precautions should be taken to prevent contamination or transmission of viruses or bacteria. I typically use hand sanitizer before the test, wear gloves, and wash my hands after administering the test. If giving the client a urine test to take to the bathroom, I always provide a paper lunch bag for added privacy. I record the result of the test in the client's chart and take a picture of the results panel for documentation.

There are many drug testing products on the market, and I have tried several with varying success. For the last several years, I have purchased my tests from Amazon. Counselors in private practice usually charge between $40 to $60 to administer a POC test in the office. I also copy the instructions and information sheet that comes with the tests and provide it to the purchaser to ensure proper use. Preferred drug tests on Amazon: 16 Panel Urine | 5 Panel Oral Fluid

Soberlink Monitoring System

Soberlink is an alcohol monitoring device I have been using since the company started. It is a highly accurate, medical-grade device that can monitor a client's blood alcohol concentration (BAC) from virtually anywhere. The Soberlink device uses facial recognition and breath technology to ensure the person using the device is the one being tested. It connects to the cellular network to upload the encrypted test result to the client's account. If the device does not have a cellular connection, it stores the tests and uploads them once a connection is re-established. It is small enough to be carried in a backpack, purse, or glove compartment and takes less than a minute to conduct a test.

The SoberSky portal provides an interface for monitoring and managing the device. You can set up custom schedules and alerts for almost any client scenario. I receive a text message and email anytime a client misses a test, fails the user authentication, or has a positive result. If a client faces legal consequences due to a positive test, misses a test, or fails authentication, I always have them take an EtG test at a laboratory to confirm whether they were drinking on the day of the test. The Soberlink device can be leased or purchased, and Soberlink has a buy-back program for purchased units that are no longer needed. Soberlink also charges a monthly monitoring fee. It is cheaper than many other monitoring options and often less expensive than frequent laboratory testing.

I have found the Soberlink device to be less invasive or obvious than other forms of monitoring such as the SCRAM bracelet or other wearable devices, with the same or better accuracy. While many professionals charge an additional monitoring fee of $50 to $150 per month on top of the Soberlink fees, I do not charge extra for regular clients as it takes very little time to monitor and I include it as part of my services. However, you are within your rights to charge an additional fee if you feel it is necessary.

Soberlink is a very effective tool for many scenarios. If a client has trouble staying sober or chronically relapses, needs additional accountability, or wants to establish trust with loved ones, it can be very effective. It is also used to monitor clients with legal situations such as criminal charges, probation, or child custody battles. Soberlink provides free training to professionals who wish to use the device in their practice, and I highly recommend taking advantage of this training.

Chapter
Twenty-Eight

SAP & SAE Training

Substance Abuse Professionals (SAP)

According to the U.S. Department of Transportation (DOT), *"transportation providers must employ workers who are 100% drug and alcohol-free."* To ensure this, the DOT developed regulations and created the position of Substance Abuse Professionals (SAPs). SAPs assist employees identified through this program as having a problem with drugs and/or alcohol or who have tested positive for drug use.

SAPs evaluate employees who have violated a DOT drug and alcohol regulation and make recommendations concerning education, treatment, follow-up testing, and continuing care. DOT regulations prevent the DOT, the Employer, or the Employee from interfering with the recommendations an SAP makes. The employee must complete all the requirements in order to return to duty.

When you evaluate an employee covered by DOT regulation as an SAP, you:

- Conduct a comprehensive face-to-face evaluation to help the employee resolve their drug or alcohol problems or prohibited drug use.

- Provide referrals to the employee based on your treatment or education requirements. SAPs may not refer employees to themselves for treatment.

- Perform in-person follow-up evaluations to ensure the employee has demonstrated successful compliance and is ready to return to duty.

- Develop a follow-up drug and alcohol testing plan to ensure continued compliance.

- Provide the employer and employee with continuing care recommendations.

Substance Abuse Expert (SAE)

The U.S. Nuclear Regulatory Commission (NRC) requires that employees at nuclear power plants and other facilities handling nuclear material are 100% drug and alcohol-free. Similar to an SAP, an SAE assists employees identified through this program as having a problem with drugs and/or alcohol or who have tested positive for drug use. SAEs perform almost identical functions and services as SAPs but for employees governed by the NRC.

Why Become an SAP or SAE?

SAPs and SAEs have the serious responsibility of protecting commercial aviation, the trucking industry, the nuclear industry, and more from serious accidents, injuries, or deaths caused by employee drug or alcohol use. Becoming an SAP or SAE allows you to generate additional income for your practice, use your skills in a critical way that ensures the safety of our country, and join a limited pool of professionals who provide these services.

I charge $1000 for SAP initial evaluations and $550 for follow-up evaluations. While this may sound high, it is often much lower than what other professionals charge for these services. Performing three or four of these evaluations per week can lead to substantial income. Similar to EAP programs, companies that manage these services for major employers often provide regular referrals to preferred SAPs.

Who is Eligible to Become an SAP or SAE?

To become a qualified SAP or SAE, you must possess one of the following credentials:
- National-level certification through the NAADAC Certification Commission for Addiction Professionals (NCC AP) or the International Certification & Reciprocity Consortium (IC&RC). Note: State-level certification does NOT meet DOT requirements.

- Master Addiction Counselors (MAC) certification through the National Board of Certified Counselors (NBCC)

- Licensed physician (Doctor of Medicine or Osteopathy)

- Licensed or certified psychologist

- Licensed or certified social worker

- Licensed or certified employee assistance professional

- Licensed or certified Marriage and Family Therapist (MFT)

In addition, you must complete a minimum of twelve hours of SAP or SAE training by a nationally recognized training organization and renew it every three years. NAADAC provides this training, while IC&RC does not. I recommend the NAADAC training program as it supports a national association for addiction professionals; however, there are other smaller training organizations available. Completing your training through NAADAC allows you to be listed in their online SAP directory. The cost for the training is $307 for NAADAC members and $407 for non-members. The price difference for members means you recoup your membership fee with this one training. NAADAC prices are competitive with other organizations.

If you have an IC&RC addiction credential, one from NAADAC, or are in one of the professions listed above, you are already qualified to take an SAP or SAE training course. You simply take the course, pass the test, receive your certificate, and begin performing the duties. While national or international certification and the SAP or SAE training can cost around $1,000, it only takes a few assessments to cover those costs. I recommend anyone who is eligible to become an SAP or SAE.

On the website, you will find comprehensive video training on how to become an SAP or SAE, what the process entails, and how to integrate it into your practice. It also covers the duties and responsibilities of SAPs and what they charge.

Chapter
Twenty-Nine

Tools, Trainings, and Certifications

B esides becoming an SAP or SAE, there are other tools, trainings, and certifications that can significantly enhance your effectiveness as a counselor and your clients' success. Some of these additional certifications can also attract more clients to your practice.

HeartMath

HeartMath is similar to biofeedback, but the equipment is very inexpensive and works with smartphones, tablets, and laptops. Clients in early recovery, and even those in sustained recovery, often struggle with sleep, staying calm, anxiety, fatigue, and depression. HeartMath uses a small electrode that connects to your finger and your device. The HeartMath app or software then guides clients through exercises to lower their heart rate and relax. Clients can also use HeartMath at home when they are not in sessions.

According to HeartMath's website (2019), a study of over 11,500 people showed improvements in mental and emotional well-being in just six to nine weeks using HeartMath training and technology:

- 24% improvement in the ability to focus

- 30% improvement in sleep

- 38% improvement in calmness

- 46% drop in anxiety

- 48% drop in fatigue

- 56% drop in depression

This training and technology can be invaluable for clients, helping to retrain their brains and improve many important areas over time. HeartMath offers free trainings for professionals and professional certification training programs. I have used HeartMath successfully with hundreds of clients and seen significant improvements in these areas. Many clients who resist yoga, meditation, or biofeedback find this solution ideal.

Certified Gambling Counselor

I do not work with gambling clients because I do not feel sufficiently trained or confident to help them. However, obtaining a Certified Gambling Counselor credential could be beneficial for your practice. There are not nearly enough Certified Gambling Counselors for those who need them. The National Council on Problem Gambling (NCPG) is a valuable resource for clients with gambling disorders.

If you go to NCPG's website and search for counselors in California, only a few clinicians are listed for a state with a population of 40 million people. By becoming a Certified Gambling Counselor, you can add your name to this list and start receiving referrals.

To become a Certified Gambling Counselor, you need specific gambling disorder training (offered by NCPG), at least 100 hours of supervised gambling disorder counseling under an approved program or clinician, and other requirements. This credential is not easy to obtain, but it fills a significant need in the community.

Motivational Interviewing

According to SAMHSA, there are multiple evidence-based behavioral therapies for substance use disorders, including Cognitive Behavioral Therapy (CBT), Motivational Enhancement Therapy (MET), Contingency Management Interventions, Community Reinforcement Approach, The Matrix Model, 12-Step Facilitation, Family Behavior Therapy, and Behavioral Therapies for Adolescents.

I have received training in Motivational Interviewing (MI) and 12-Step Facilitation. MI, developed by clinical psychologists William Miller and Stephen Rollnick, is particularly effective in resolving ambivalence in clients appropriate for outpatient counseling. MI is a directive, client-centered counseling approach that elicits behavioral change by helping clients resolve ambivalence.

Learning and implementing MI has made me more effective as a counselor. Unfortunately, many schools do not properly inform students about this evidence-based treatment or teach them how to use it. I highly suggest reading the bestselling "Motivational Interviewing:

Helping People Change (3rd Edition)" and taking an in-person MI training course. An organization called MINT provides trainings and connects providers.

Hypnotherapy

While I am not a hypnotherapist, hypnotherapy might be helpful for some of your clients. I became interested in hypnotherapy after learning that the Giants Manager Bruce Bochy and others quit their long-term chewing tobacco habit after a single session. Hypnotherapy can be a powerful tool for overcoming addictions and other issues.

While hypnotherapy may not work for everyone, it could be an effective intervention for some clients. Different clients may need different interventions and techniques to be successful, and hypnotherapy can be one of those options.

Employee Assistance Programs (EAP)

There are hundreds of EAPs around the country that contract with employers to provide various services to employees, including confidential assistance with substance abuse problems. EAPs typically refer clients for assessments and counseling sessions, preauthorizing a certain number of sessions, usually between two and six, and compensating you at a predetermined rate per session.

While the average payment for sessions is $60 per visit (sometimes as high as $90 for PhD-level clinicians), whether this rate is acceptable depends on your practice. If your practice is busy, taking clients at this reduced rate may impact your earnings significantly. However, if this rate would improve your earnings or bolster your caseload, then accepting EAP clients is beneficial. EAP clients often convert to regular clients once the EAP stops covering sessions.

To find EAP companies, simply search for "EAP companies" online, visit their websites, and look for a page about becoming a provider. I have compiled a list of EAP companies I have worked with and had good experiences with on the website.

A Rational Workbook for Change-2nd Edition

My friend and colleague, Dr. John Herdman, has written a workbook for clients called *A Rational Workbook for Change-2nd Edition*. This workbook implements evidence-based cognitive-behavioral therapy concepts to help clients change their thoughts, feelings, and behaviors.

Chapter Thirty

A Final Word, Not Goodbye

This is not a goodbye, but a welcome! Welcome to the growing community of behavioral health professionals providing these critical services in private practice. I hope that everyone who has read this book has developed a deep understanding of the responsibility we have as addiction professionals in private practice. Throughout my career, I have taken these responsibilities seriously and have worked hard to uphold them. I have always understood that I don't just represent myself—I represent our entire profession. This realization drives me to provide the most professional and effective services possible to my clients.

We are in a period of incredible change in our industry and profession. Research continues to refine our understanding of what is effective and what is not. I urge you to remain open-minded to these developments and always remember that what helped you or other clients may differ greatly from what will help others. It is an exciting time to be behavioral health professional and to participate in the paradigm shift occurring in our field. We are at the forefront of effecting positive change for those suffering from substance use disorders, not only with our clients but also at the local, state, and national levels.

You represent our profession. Remember this in everything you do. As laws and regulations evolve, we should inspire these changes, not be the reason for them. When I first started in private practice, I had very little specific information related to the best practices of an addiction counselor. I investigated how other professionals and disciplines managed these issues in their fields and adapted them to create the model I use for my practice. Please investigate best practices and consult when you come across issues you haven't previously encountered. Before you launch your practice, there is no better time to complete the required ethics training for recertification or licensing.

Please email me or join the conversation and community I have created to propel us forward. You don't need to do this alone. Let's keep growing and succeeding together; please join me at AddictionP rivatePractice.com.

Thank you! May you exceed the success I have experienced and change the world one session at a time.

Chapter Thirty-One

Telehealth

The advent of telehealth has revolutionized the field of behavioral health, offering unprecedented access to care for clients and flexibility for providers. For addiction counselors, integrating telehealth into a private practice can enhance service delivery, improve client engagement, and extend reach to underserved populations. It can also expand your pool of potential clients from your local area to the entire state. This chapter provides a comprehensive guide to incorporating telehealth into your practice, covering legal and ethical considerations, technology requirements, best practices for virtual sessions, and strategies for maintaining client rapport and therapeutic effectiveness.

What is Telehealth?

Telehealth is commonly accepted as services delivered via telephone or video. Some online platforms use an internet-based chat/text interface and email as part of their telehealth services.

Many counselors prefer in-person sessions over the idea of telehealth, often without having tried it. The COVID-19 pandemic created a radical acceptance of telehealth, and many clients now prefer it over in-person visits. Concerns about detecting relapses without seeing the entire body or smelling alcohol are often unfounded. Even with phone sessions, counselors can become attuned to a client's voice, detecting changes that indicate substance use.

State Regulations

Before offering telehealth services, ensure compliance with state regulations. Each state has different rules regarding telehealth, including requirements for cross-state practice and the necessity of holding a license or certification in the client's or provider's state of residence. While telehealth is legal in all 50 states, some states require additional steps, such as confirming the client's physical location before starting the session and documenting it in your progress notes.

Confidentiality and Privacy

Maintaining client confidentiality is paramount. Use HIPAA-compliant platforms for video conferencing and secure electronic health records (EHR). Inform clients about privacy measures and obtain their consent for telehealth services. This also applies to ensuring that no one can overhear sessions through open windows, doors, or thin walls.

Informed Consent

Create a telehealth-specific informed consent form. This document should outline the nature of telehealth services, potential risks and benefits, confidentiality limits, and emergency protocols. Discuss this consent form with clients before beginning telehealth sessions to ensure they understand and agree to the terms. A free telehealth consent form is available on my website AddictionPrivatePractice.com.

Choosing the Right Platform

Select a reliable, user-friendly telehealth platform that complies with HIPAA regulations. Platforms like Zoom for Healthcare or Microsoft Teams are popular choices, as many clients use them in their daily lives. Evaluate features such as video quality, ease of use, integration with EHR systems, and cost. If you use an EHR platform like SimplePractice, it includes a free HIPAA-compliant video interface, so you don't need an additional subscription for Zoom or Teams.

Equipment and Setup

Invest in high-quality equipment to ensure a professional experience. This includes a computer or tablet with a good camera and microphone, a stable internet connection, and appropriate lighting. Encourage clients to also find a quiet, private space for their sessions.

Technical Support

Offer technical support for clients who may be unfamiliar with telehealth technology. Provide clear instructions for accessing the platform and consider having a test session to troubleshoot any issues before the first official appointment.

Establishing the Right Environment

Create a professional and comfortable environment for your tele-health sessions. Ensure your background is clean and uncluttered and maintain eye contact by looking into the camera. Encourage clients to find a private and quiet space free from distractions. Ensure that no one can hear your sessions through an open window or door that isn't soundproof. Often, just putting a noise maker outside your home office door does the trick. Do not allow your clients to drive or engage in any other distracting activity while you are in session. Ask them to pull over so that they can participate in the sessions safely.

Building and Maintaining Rapport

Building rapport in a virtual setting can be challenging but is essential. Use active listening and verbal affirmations to show empathy and understanding. Pay attention to non-verbal cues and encourage clients to express themselves fully. Be patient and give clients time to adjust to the telehealth format.

Engagement Techniques

Incorporate interactive tools to keep clients engaged. Use screen sharing for educational materials, digital whiteboards for exercises, and secure messaging for between-session communication. Encourage clients to take part actively and set clear goals for each session.

Assessment and Treatment Planning

Adapt your assessment tools and treatment plans for the virtual environment. Use validated online assessment tools and questionnaires. Collaborate with clients to develop realistic and achievable treatment goals, considering the telehealth format. Almost every tool we use in private practice is now online and cloud-based, including assessment tools like those found at Herdman Health.

Crisis Management

Have a clear crisis management plan in place. Know the local resources in the client's area, including emergency contacts and mental health crisis services. Ensure clients know how to reach you in case of an emergency and establish a protocol for handling crises during a telehealth session. You should ask your client for their physical location at the start of every session and document that location in your notes.

Insurance and Reimbursement Policies

If you accept insurance, familiarize yourself with insurance policies regarding telehealth. Many insurers cover telehealth services, but the extent of coverage can vary. Verify coverage with each client's insurance provider and understand the billing codes and documentation requirements for telehealth services. You will often use the same service code, but add a modifier code to show that the session was conducted via telehealth.

Setting Fees

Your fees for telehealth services should be the same as they are for in-person sessions. You do not need to lower your fee for telehealth services. If your practice is 100% telehealth and that substantially reduces your overhead expenses, you can always decide to adjust your fees accordingly in the future.

Documentation

Maintain thorough records of all telehealth sessions. Document session content, client progress, their location, and any technical issues encountered. Be sure that the client is in a stationary and private environment in your documentation.

Integrating telehealth into your addiction private practice can significantly enhance your ability to provide flexible, accessible, and effective care. By understanding the legal and ethical considerations, investing in the right technology, implementing best practices for virtual sessions, and staying informed about billing and reimbursement policies, you can successfully transition to a telehealth model. Embrace the opportunities that telehealth offers to expand your reach and continue making a positive impact on the lives of your clients.

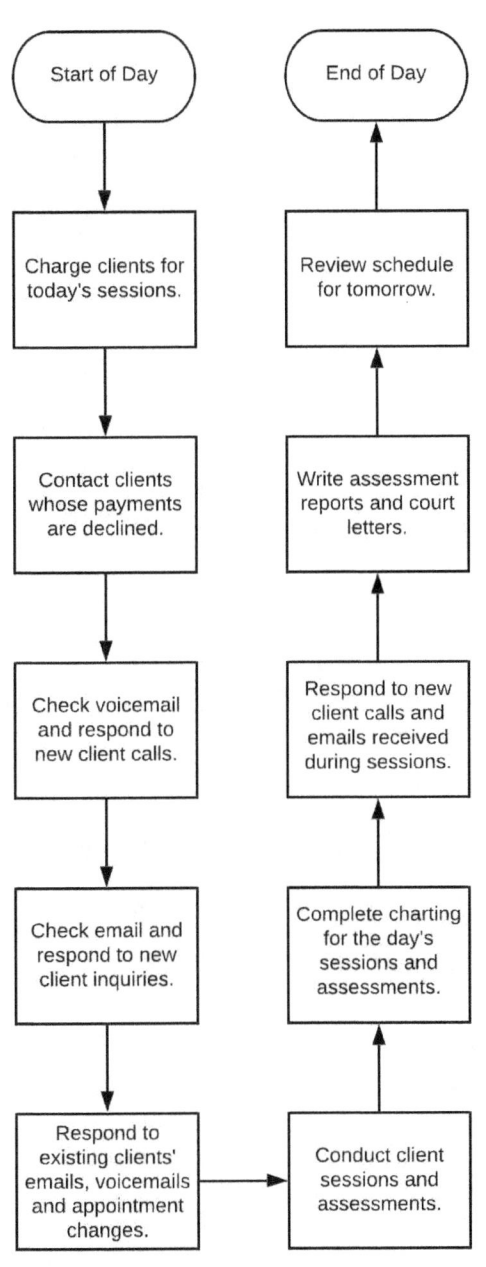

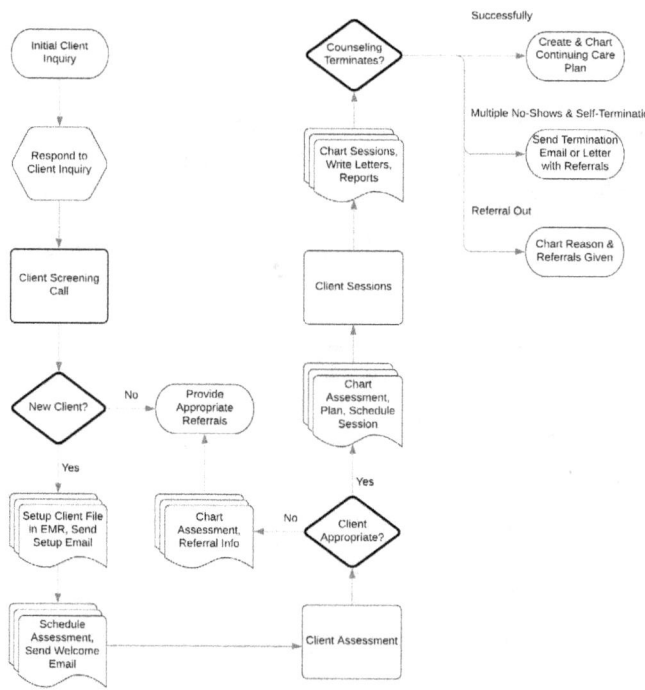

Initial Client Inquiry

Respond to Client Inquiry

Client Screening Call

New Client? — No → Provide Appropriate Referrals

Yes

Setup Client File in EMR, Send Setup Email

Chart Assessment, Referral Info

Schedule Assessment, Send Welcome Email

Client Assessment

Client Appropriate? — No → Chart Assessment, Referral Info

Yes

Chart Assessment, Plan, Schedule Session

Client Sessions

Chart Sessions, Write Letters, Reports

Counseling Terminates?

Successfully → Create & Chart Continuing Care Plan

Multiple No-Shows & Self-Termination → Send Termination Email or Letter with Referrals

Referral Out → Chart Reason & Referrals Given

Chapter Thirty-Two

Everyone's Biggest Fears

After several years in private practice, I've noticed that most counselors encounter similar fears when starting their own business. Imposter syndrome is also a common feeling among providers, and it's completely normal. If you weren't nervous about at least one aspect of launching your own business, I would be concerned.

When I first started private practice over a decade ago, only a few brave addiction counselors were doing the same across the country. There were no guides, classes, best practices, or tools—I was completely on my own. I made countless mistakes, tried various tools and software programs, and experimented with different marketing strategies, most of which didn't work and cost me a lot of money. You have the benefit of launching your business without making those mistakes. My pain will become your success, and I'm excited for you!

The biggest fears include:

· Building a website

· Writing content for their website

· Writing their online profile text

· Having enough clients

· Lawsuits

· Paying taxes

· Asking clients for payments

Does that list seem accurate? You may have found some new things to be anxious about that you hadn't even thought about before – sorry! The first step is to adopt an adventure mindset to replace anxiety. Remember when you were in college and took a course that excited you? You looked forward to each lesson with fascination. One of those classes for me was Psychopharmacology.

You are embarking on a new adventure, just like when you went to school to become a behavioral health professional. If you could do that, you can absolutely do this. I am here to help you along the way and provide the support you need to be successful. If you haven't already done so, visit AddictionPrivatePractice.com and explore all the support options available to you!

Let me break down how I can help you with each area and explain how we will overcome these fears.

Building a Website

What I hope you learned from the website section of this book is that you don't need to overthink your website. You only need the few pages and the content I described. However, I realize that setting up the website and writing the text can be overwhelming.

You'll find incredible AI-powered resources on Wix.com or Go-Daddy that allow you to easily create a clean, professional, and inexpensive website. I also offer a website development package on Ad dictionPrivatePractice.com that is affordable, with payment options available.

Once your website is complete, the hard part is over. You will only need to update it when you make changes to your practice that new clients need to know about.

Writing Content for Your Website

Writing content is often the biggest roadblock to completing a website or other marketing tools. In the first edition of my book, I created worksheets to help you create content by following simple instructions. Those are still available to you on my website. Now, we have gone a step further to make this even simpler. I have developed a software tool that allows you to answer some questions, and it produces your website content for you! It will take your information and generate perfectly worded content for your web pages. You can modify the text as needed and then cut and paste it into your website.

Writing Your Online Profile Text

Most counselors experience the same problem with writing their profile text. Online directories often limit the amount of text you can include in your profile, requiring you to fit critical information into a limited number of characters. My software tool writes all the text for you, personalized to your strengths and specializations, and fits it into the required space allowance. This allows you to have a world-class, honest profile that attracts appropriate clients immediately.

Enrolling Enough Clients

You cannot succeed in private practice and achieve financial independence without clients. If you follow and implement the basic marketing activities outlined in this book, you will attract clients. However, I have developed a marketing strategy over the past 10 years that anyone can employ and start receiving a steady stream of clients quickly. This strategy is too valuable to include in this book. I guarantee this method and course—if you don't feel it brings you new clients quickly, I'll refund your course fee. It is inexpensive and easy to implement—visit AddictionPrivatePractice.com to learn more about this advanced marketing course today. You won't regret it.

Lawsuits

Getting sued by a client is our worst nightmare. While it has never happened to me or any of my colleagues in private practice, it can happen. I believe that if you provide compassionate, evidence-based (MI, CBT), and highly ethical services, your chances of being sued are very small. Typically, it is major violations of ethics, like having a relationship with a client or breaking confidentiality, that lead to lawsuits.

The good news is that malpractice insurance protects you in the event of a lawsuit. The insurance company will hire and pay an attorney to defend you, and they will also pay a settlement up to the value of the policy. Most attorneys who defend these cases are experienced and often settle out of court for an amount well below your policy maximum to avoid a costly court battle.

Self-Employment Taxes

Many counselors say they don't go into private practice because they don't want to pay additional self-employment taxes. This argument is ridiculous. Yes, you will pay more taxes if you earn substantially more, but the increase in income is well worth the extra tax. You will also need to pay self-employment tax, which is simply the portion of payroll taxes an employer would normally cover. It's not a large amount of your new income. If you are employed, your employer is paying those taxes, which you will assume if you earn money in private practice.

Don't let the fear of additional taxes hold you back from financial freedom. Paying more taxes is a quality problem—it means you are making more money. Here is one more important benefit to owning your own business – everything you spend on that business is also tax deductible. This often means you pay fewer taxes than if you worked for an employer.

Asking Clients for Payments

Some providers find it difficult to ask for and collect money from their clients. If you worked at a program where finances were always handled by someone else, this can be uncomfortable at first, but you will get used to it. Your clients are entering a business relationship with you and expect to pay your fees. No one thinks counselors can do this for free, and often clients are happy to pay you and feel good when they do. If this issue seriously bothers you, you may need to work on codependency. Just as you don't go to the doctor, dentist, or massage therapist expecting free services, your clients won't either.

The system I described in this book of charging clients each morning before you come into the office is an excellent way of handling your billing while having fewer tough conversations.

By adopting an adventure mindset, leveraging available resources, and addressing your fears head-on, you can successfully navigate the challenges of starting your private practice. Remember, you are not alone on this journey. With the right tools and support, you can achieve your goals and make a positive impact on the lives of your clients.